CMA
Study Guide

Ace the Certified Medical Assistant Exam on Your First Try with No Effort | Test Questions, Answer Keys & Insider Tips to Score a 98% Pass Rate

Craig MacMillan

Table of Contents

CHAPTER 3: CLINICAL COMPETENCY _____ 23

Introduction

A must-have for anyone hoping to earn their CMA credential in the near future, "Certified Medical Assistant Study Guide" covers every topic on the CMA exam in exhaustive detail. This updated edition covers all the necessary topics required to become a certified medical assistant, including clinical competency, general administrative knowledge, legal and ethical issues, and medication administration.

The book starts with an introduction that provides an overview of the CMA exam and the eligibility requirements. It then proceeds to cover the registration and application process, scheduling an exam, retake policies, and what to expect on exam day.

The second chapter provides valuable tips on how to pass the CMA exam, including strategies to overcome test anxiety and effective study techniques.

The third chapter delves into clinical competency, which is a critical component of a medical assistant's role. It covers patient intake and discharge, medical terminology, vital signs, patient interviewing and documentation, infection control, emergency management, and an overview of the body systems and their functions. The chapter also includes a section on medication administration, which covers various types of drugs, preparation, and administration.

The fourth chapter covers general administrative knowledge, including legal and ethical issues, communication skills, and scheduling appointments. It also includes a section on billing, coding, and insurance.

Chapter 6 focuses on preparing for the Certified Emergency Nurse (CEN) exam, which is a specialized certification for emergency nurses. This chapter provides test-taking tips, study strategies, and an overview of the exam.

Chapter 7 provides sample questions to test the reader's knowledge and understanding of the material covered in the book, while chapter 8 offers detailed explanations and answers to those questions.

Finally, the book includes a bonus chapter that offers three secret keys to success in the CMA exam, including planning effectively, studying productively, and practicing the right way.

Chapter 1

The CMA Exam

It can be both tough and rewarding to work toward becoming a Certified Medical Assistant (CMA). The complexity and range of duties for medical assistants increase along with the healthcare sector's evolution. You are making a commitment to clinical competence and patient care by pursuing CMA certification, not just accepting a position.

However, there is a significant obstacle you must overcome before donning your white coat and joining the ranks of healthcare professionals: the CMA test. This test is more than just a collection of questions; it's a thorough evaluation meant to determine how prepared you are to work in a medical setting. It checks how well you understand fundamental clinical, administrative, and general healthcare concepts and makes sure you're prepared for the varied requirements of the work.

You're not alone if you're experiencing a mix of excitement and apprehension at this moment. This chapter tries to guide you through the frequently complex landscape of the CMA test, which many others before you have encountered at this critical juncture in their professional journeys. From comprehending the eligibility requirements to making sense of the score system, we'll be breaking through the entire procedure. We'll walk you through the specifics of the application process, exam scheduling, costs, and other logistical considerations that might seem difficult but are necessary for a seamless experience.

Consider this chapter to be your dependable road map. It gives structured information, allowing you to quickly find what you need, much like a neatly arranged medical chart. We've got you covered, whether you're interested in the retake procedures or are already dreading what exam day might entail.

Eligibility Requirements

The American Association of Medical Assistants (AAMA) administers the Certified Medical Assistant (CMA) certification, a respected credential in the healthcare sector. This certification validates a candidate's competence in duties that are essential to efficient patient care and healthcare operations on both a clinical and administrative level. Candidates must meet specific requirements in order to take the CMA exam.

Education Requirements

Candidates for the CMA exam must have finished a medical assisting program that has been approved by the Accrediting Bureau of Health Education Schools (ABHES) or the Commission on Accreditation of Allied Health Education Programs (CAAHEP). These courses normally last one to two years to complete and combine classroom learning with real-world experience. Essential subjects in patient care, clinical practices, and administrative duties should all be included in the training.

Professional Certification Requirements

Medical assistants can only be certified through the CMA exam. As a result, you cannot take the CMA exam if you hold a different qualification, such as Registered Nurse (RN) or Licensed Practical Nurse (LPN). To achieve the requirements for this particular certification, you must complete a medical assisting program from an authorized college.

Experience Requirements

While the educational component is usually the focus, some candidates could be curious about work experience. Completing the recognized educational program is typically thought to be sufficient for eligibility for the CMA test. In other words, standardized schooling is prioritized over inconsistent work experience. The experience you gain from an internship or externship, which is frequently a component of an accredited educational program, will help you in both the exam and in your future profession.

According to the American Association of Medical Assistants (AAMA), a Certified Medical Assistant is someone "who performs both administrative and clinical tasks in medical offices, clinics, and other healthcare facilities." The breadth of tasks performed by a CMA includes everything from gathering patient histories and getting them ready for tests to carrying out quick clinical procedures and handling front-desk duties.

Verification Requirements:

All applicants seeking to become Certified Medical Assistants have their credentials and qualifications carefully checked by the American Association of Medical Assistants (AAMA). In light of this, documentation is a crucial component of the verification procedure.

Educational Documentation

Candidates must offer certified transcripts from the college or university where they finished a recognized program for medical assistance. These transcripts should list the program's accreditation status and include information about the courses taken. Typically, transcripts are given to the AAMA directly from the educational institution.

Professional Experience Documentation

The emphasis here is less on professional experience and more on education because passing an authorized program is the primary requirement for eligibility for the CMA exam. Any internship or externship you complete as part of your academic program, however, should be documented. This frequently takes the form of an official certificate or letter of completion from the program, which must also be presented to the AAMA for verification.

Additional Verification

The AAMA reserves the right to make contact with academic institutions or externship or internship sites for additional verification, even if this is uncommon. This can entail verifying participation, course completion, and the caliber and content of the training you got.

The AAMA mandates that candidates go through this extensive verification process in order to uphold the credibility and high standards connected with the CMA certification. Before submitting their applications to take the exam, prospective CMAs should carefully consider these requirements.

In the medical field, the Certified Medical Assistant credential is a sign of dedication and professionalism. Being eligible and making it through the verification process are the first and most important steps in obtaining this prestigious certification.

How to Register for the Exam

When you have a map in your hands, navigating the registration maze for any certification exam becomes much less terrifying. If you know what to anticipate, pursuing the American Association of Medical Assistants' (AAMA) Certified Medical Assistant (CMA) certification is a rather simple process. Let's now reveal this map to you.

Application

Candidates must first register for an account on the AAMA website, which serves as the entrance to the online application. You can view the detailed application form that requests a variety of personal information once your account is ready. You'll need to carefully fill out the information regarding your school background and any relevant employment experience, not merely check the appropriate boxes. These are necessary for the AAMA to determine whether you are qualified to take the CMA exam.

Notification

Hold tight after submitting your application. You will receive an email from the AAMA confirming receipt of your application. This email will not only act as a virtual pat on the back, but it will also direct you through the next several steps. It will mostly include information on the supporting papers required to confirm your eligibility, such as transcripts, potential certificates, and proof of any necessary job or internship experience.

Approval

At this point, patience is a virtue. After receiving the necessary paperwork from you, the AAMA will begin a verification process that could take up to three weeks. You'll get another email with a golden ticket—the authorization to schedule your exam—if the planets are in the right alignment and your application is accepted.

Scheduling an Exam

Prometric collaborates with the AAMA as its testing partner. To choose a comfortable location and establish an actual exam date, you must visit the Prometric website. Finding a nearby site should be simple given Prometric's vast network of test facilities.

Rescheduling an Exam

Again, Prometric's website is your best bet if you find yourself in a predicament where you need to reschedule. But remember, rescheduling isn't a casual process. There are due dates and possible costs, so it's wise to familiarize yourself with this information beforehand.

Application Fees

The real action begins right here. Application for the CMA exam is not inexpensive. Whether you are an AAMA member or not affects how much you pay. Additionally, be prepared to pay more money if you need to change your appointment time or receive more score reports.

Retake Policies

Even the strongest falter. You are not out of the running if you don't pass the exam on your first try. The AAMA permits retakes, but only in certain circumstances. Before you may try again, a time period must pass, and yes, there will be a fee. Review these conditions in order to avoid being surprised.

Now that you have the essentials, you can proceed with the CMA exam registration process. Each of the aforementioned processes has its own patterns and guidelines: application, notice, approval, scheduling, and even contingencies like rescheduling and retests. Exam preparation involves more than simply studying; it also involves understanding the procedures that will get you to the testing facility.

What to Expect on Exam Day

The day of the exam is frequently the climax of weeks, months, or even years of study. But you don't want any unpleasant shocks. Knowing what to anticipate can help make the exam experience less stressful while also calming any anxiety. So let's explore the Certified Medical Assistant (CMA) Exam's world.

What to Do

Arrive early—at least 30 minutes prior to the exam's planned start time. You must have proper identification with you in order to enter the testing facility. Since only necessary objects that have been permitted by the exam may be brought into the testing room, most facilities will offer a designated place for personal goods.

Mode of Exam Delivery

The CMA test is given in a proctored setting and is computer-based. Even if you have computer experience, keep in mind that different exam software can have a variety of interfaces. To eliminate any hiccups, it would be advantageous to become familiar with standard computer-based testing techniques.

Exam Length

The CMA exam is more like a well-paced marathon than a sprint. Over the course of 160 minutes, you will see a total of 160 questions. Four segments of 40 questions each are created from these questions. Time management is, you guessed it, essential.

Exam Breaks

The good news is that while there are optional brief intermissions between segments, the clock does not run. These are quick chances to move around, breathe, and collect your thoughts. Never undervalue the restorative impact of a quick break; it can mean the difference in those final 40 questions.

Exam Format

Each multiple-choice question on the exam has four potential solutions. In addition to having the necessary knowledge, reading each question thoroughly is essential for success. A regrettable but preventable blunder can be the failure to understand a question.

How Exams are Scored

A scaled scoring system is used for the CMA exam. Out of the 160 questions, 200 are scored, while the remaining 20 are practice questions for upcoming tests and do not count toward your final grade. Scores range from 0 to 600, with 430 serving as the cutoff. But don't be fooled by the figures; the exam is difficult, and each question is important.

Rules and Regulations

There will be a tight rule of conduct at the testing facility because this isn't the Wild West. Be prepared for security cameras and perhaps a one-on-one proctor. The use of dishonest methods will automatically disqualify you. In general, personal items like phones, watches, and notes are not permitted in the examination room. To avoid tension at the last minute, be aware of the guidelines in advance.

Getting Test Results

Tense as if you want to bite your nails, right? Normally, your preliminary results are available right away following the test, however they are not your final results. Within eight weeks, the AAMA will normally publish the official findings. This extra time enables rigorous examination results analysis and statistical equivalence methods to guarantee fairness and correctness.

You now have it. Your exam day's anatomy will be exposed and dissected. Nearly as important as understanding the exam subject itself can be knowing what to anticipate and how to deal with the complications of the exam day. You are prepared for a full experience, not simply for questions that will appear on a screen.

Chapter 2

How To Pass The CMA Exam

Your strategy room is Chapter 2, the central location where we'll talk about how to succeed on the Certified Medical Assistant (CMA) Exam rather than just get by. Understanding the subject matter and exam style isn't sufficient; you also need to be adept in high-stakes testing psychology and techniques. This chapter will explore the art of test-taking by exploring useful advice, methods for reducing test anxiety, and efficient study practices.

We start with "Test Tips," which are the strategic steps to mastering exam problems. We'll then address the proverbial elephant in the room: test anxiety. It affects even the sharpest minds and is more common than you might imagine. We'll offer you practical guidance to help you regain mental control. The "Study Strategy," a comprehensive approach to take in, hold onto, and remember everything you need to know, will round up our discussion.

Test Tips

In order to succeed on the Certified Medical Assistant (CMA) exam, one must not only study extensively but learn about all the tips they can get their hands on and put them to good use. Here are a few of the tips that may come in handy for passing the CMA exam.

Understanding Question Types

There are many different types of questions on the CMA exam. Knowing what to expect can be half the battle when it comes to multiple-choice and scenario-based things. To get a feel for the kinds of questions you'll see on the test, look at previous exams or practice tests.

Time Management

You can either use the clock as an ally or a foe. Spending too much time on challenging questions and rushing through the simpler ones is a classic rookie error. Use pacing to your advantage. Set up definite time periods and stick to them for groups of questions.

Elimination Method

Don't just skip over difficult questions when you don't know the answer off the top of your head. Use the elimination process. There are frequently one or two solutions out of the four or five that are obviously incorrect. In order to improve your chances of picking the right response, discard them first.

Prioritize Scenarios

Scenario-based questions are time-consuming in addition to being difficult. You typically have to deal with situational challenges. When your brain is at its sharpest, address issues early so you can read, analyze, and respond quickly.

Utilize All Available Resources

Use footnotes, graphs, and charts in addition to the main text when responding to queries. Sometimes, especially in issues that strongly rely on interpretation or situational analysis, these auxiliary elements can provide knowledge that leads to the right response.

Double-Check Before Submission

If time allows after finishing, go back and check your responses. A question is simple to mistake or misunderstand when you first read it. Use this time to correct any errors and make sure your decisions are sound.

Practical Skill Application

Keep in mind that the CMA Exam assesses your practical application of knowledge, not simply your academic comprehension. When responding to questions, evaluate how the information works in a practical situation as well as what it says in the book.

Trust Your Gut

Your initial reaction may not always be the best one. It might be a good idea to believe your gut if you're torn between two options and have an opinion about one of them, unless there is compelling proof to the contrary.

By combining these test-taking strategies into your exam strategy, you're equipping yourself with a mental toolkit made specifically for the CMA Exam: a triumphant performance. With these tactics at your disposal, you're one step closer to wearing your CMA certification as a badge of honor.

How To Overcome Test Anxiety

Many people suffer anxiety when studying for and taking professional exams like the Certified Medical Assistant (CMA) exam. Anxiety, or the experience of anxiousness, anticipation, or worry about taking an examination, can have a detrimental effect on test performance. However, there are a number of methods available to help test-takers calm their nerves and perform to their full potential on the CMA exam.

Recognize the Signs

Recognizing its onset is the first step in treating test anxiety. The symptoms can include a fast heartbeat, perspiration, trembling, and even lightheadedness. You can use coping mechanisms when you have a basic understanding of how your body responds.

Implement Mindfulness Techniques

The benefits of centering yourself when worry sets in can't be overstated. Your neural system can be reset by methods like focused breathing, which involves taking a deep breath in via your nose, holding it for a short period of time, and then exhaling through your mouth. By keeping you focused on the now, mindfulness successfully reduces anxiety, which is typically caused by worrying about what may happen in the future.

Lean on Support Networks

Exam stress management tips and emotional support can be obtained from friends, family, or even mentors. Talking about your concerns can occasionally help them seem less overwhelming. You might also learn fresh tactics from an outside perspective that you hadn't thought of.

Active Study Methods

The lack of effectiveness of passive reading and mechanical memory can make anxiety symptoms worse. Use active learning strategies instead, such as interactive applications, flashcards, or practice tests. There is less room for anxiety the better prepared you are.

Organize and Plan

Stress can be reduced by creating a thorough study schedule weeks before the exam. Establish a schedule, allot time for each part, and know what needs to be addressed. The satisfaction of marking off areas that have been finished can act as a positive reinforcement, which naturally lowers tension.

Stay Physically Active

The body's natural mood enhancers, endorphins, are released during physical activity. Even 20 minutes of light exercise can reduce anxiety for several hours. Maintaining physical activity, whether it's a fast workout at the gym, a brisk stroll, or a jog, helps you efficiently manage stress.

Professional Help

Consider seeking professional assistance if your anxiety is so bad that it significantly impairs your ability to study or take exams. Your needs-specific coping methods can be provided by counselors or therapists. In severe circumstances, some could even recommend medication.

Visualize Success

Before entering the exam room, close your eyes for a moment and picture yourself passing the test and getting a good grade. This positive reinforcement can help you feel more confident before the challenging task that lies ahead.

Avoid Last-Minute Cramming

Tension is frequently high in the moments leading up to entering the exam room. Even though it could be alluring, preparing for an exam at the last minute can make you forget things and make you more anxious. Instead, use this opportunity to relax by taking deep breaths.

Embrace the Challenge

Finally, rather than viewing the exam as a danger to your self-worth, reframe it as a task you can overcome. This change in viewpoint could significantly impact how you approach the exam and handle anxiety.

It's similar to negotiating a challenging labyrinth to find your way through the maze of test anxiety. It necessitates a variety of coping skills, emotional intelligence, and strategic thinking. By using these techniques, you may take the initiative back from test fear and create a performance that accurately reflects your ability.

Study Strategy

The key to success on the CMA exam is developing an effective study plan. If you want to study smarter, follow these guidelines:

Know Your Syllabus

It's crucial to know what's on the table before diving into your studies. Learn everything on the course syllabus. Divide it into parts or units so you can see exactly what has to be done. You will use this road map as a reference to help you plan your time and resources more effectively.

Create a Study Calendar

Create a study schedule after you have a breakdown of your course. Set out days or weeks for each section, taking into account the time needed for practice tests and study. Put this calendar where it will be seen and follow it as carefully as you can.

Active Learning Over Passive Reading

It's simple to read a textbook and think you understand something. However, active learning, which involves using more of your senses and cognitive abilities, can greatly improve information retention. Use strategies like explaining topics to someone else, summarizing chapters in your own words, or even holding a mock class.

Variety is the Spice of Study

Increase the variety of your study materials to avoid boredom or fatigue. Don't restrict yourself to reading textbooks. Make use of discussion forums, interactive apps, video lectures, and online courses. Different formats can present various viewpoints, broadening and strengthening your learning.

Practice Makes Perfect

Practice exams and exam papers from prior years are troves of knowledge. They can aid you in comprehending the format, level of difficulty, and nature of the questions you can anticipate on the exam. As you progress, keep track of your scores and focus on improving your weak areas until they are strong.

Chunking Method

Separate your reading material into digestible sections. According to research, shorter, more focused study periods help our brains retain information better than longer ones. The Pomodoro Technique, which involves small rests in between tasks, can help your brain relax and regenerate.

Study Groups and Peer Reviews

Working with peers might provide you with insights on areas you might have missed. Studying becomes more interesting when there is a social component added. But be selective in the group you choose. To avoid such sessions becoming ineffective, they should share your motivation.

Self-Assessment

Assess yourself periodically to determine where you stand. This might take the shape of brief tests, chapter summaries, or even one-on-one tutorials. Self-evaluation identifies areas that may require more focus in addition to reinforcing what you have already learnt.

Mnemonic Techniques

Mnemonic devices can be helpful for information or sequences that are difficult to remember. To make it easier to remember complex material, make an acronym, utilize rhyming words, or even compose a brief story.

Nutrition and Rest

Although it may sound cliched, a balanced diet and enough sleep are important for improving cognitive abilities. Your brain is an organ that requires nutrition and rest in order to function at its best.

Using a planned approach to your research can make what initially seems like an impossible effort bearable and even pleasant. Your chances of passing the CMA Exam with flying colors can be significantly increased by developing a study plan that is tailored to your learning preferences and time limits. It's similar like getting ready for a lengthy journey: with the correct map, equipment, and attitude, you're far more likely to arrive at your destination safely.

Chapter 3

Clinical Competency

T he third chapter is devoted to clinical competency, an essential part of any healthcare provider's job description. Patient intake and discharge, medical terminology, interviewing patients, safety and infection control, emergency management, risk management, quality assurance, and reporting of patient safety variances are all discussed in this chapter. An summary of the anatomy, physiology, and functions of the various body systems is also included in this chapter. It also includes information on vaccines, drug classifications, and how to properly prepare and give both oral and parenteral drugs.

The objective of this chapter is to give medical personnel a thorough grounding in clinical workflow, safety, and infection control practices, patient care, and drug administration. With more information and practice, they should be able to better care for patients and make fewer mistakes. In addition, the chapter covers a variety of subjects to provide healthcare professionals with the tools they need to succeed in a variety of clinical settings.

If you're a healthcare professional interested in increasing your clinical competence and keeping up with the newest medical developments, this chapter is a great place to start! It stresses the significance of providing safe, high-quality care to patients in accordance with established practices and norms. Care for patients, patient safety, medication management, and emergency procedures are just few of the many aspects of clinical competency that are discussed in this chapter.

Clinical Workflow: Patient Intake and Discharge

Clinical competence for medical assistants includes knowledge of the patient intake and discharge process. Both the patient's initial check-in and final exit from the medical center are part of this process. The medical assistant takes down patient information such as name, address, insurance, and purpose for visit during the intake procedure. The medical assistant is responsible for ensuring that the patient has completed all required paperwork, including those related to insurance and HIPAA.

Vital Signs

In order to assess a patient's health, vital signs are essential. Assistants in medicine should be able to take accurate readings of a variety of vitals, including blood pressure, pulse, respiration rate, and temperature. A medical assistant's ability to record accurate vital sign readings is also crucial.

Medical Terminology

In the healthcare field, a specific vocabulary known as "medical terminology" is utilized. A working knowledge of anatomy, physiology, pathology, and medical procedures is essential for medical assistants. They also need to know how to interpret and use medical jargon and acronyms seen in patient charts.

Patient Interviewing Techniques and Documentation

The ability to effectively interview patients is a must for every medical assistant. They need to have good communication skills so that they can ask patients the right questions and learn about the patient's symptoms, medical history, and current medications. Medical assistants also have the responsibility of accurately recording the results of patient interviews in their patients' medical records.

Patient Screenings/Wellness Assessments

Checkups and other health evaluations of patients are essential parts of preventative medicine. Screenings and evaluations, such as those for vision, hearing, blood sugar, and cholesterol, are only some of the duties that fall under the purview of a medical assistant. They also need to know how to operate the numerous pieces of testing equipment that are at their disposal.

Processing Provider Orders

When it comes to fulfilling physician orders, medical assistants need to know the ins and outs. This involves receiving and checking orders, following up on orders that are missing information or are erroneous, and completing any paperwork that may be required.

Medical assistants must possess a comprehensive understanding of several domains, encompassing patient intake and discharge protocols, measurement of vital signs, medical terminology, interviewing strategies, documentation practices, patient screenings, wellness assessments, and order management. These abilities are crucial to patient care and to the smooth running of healthcare institutions.

Safety and Infection Control

In healthcare, safety and prevention of infection are of paramount importance. Healthcare providers, in order to protect their patients, must be aware of the dangers posed by various infectious agents and diseases. With this information, they can take the necessary precautions to stop the spread of disease.

Infectious agents

Microorganisms that can cause illness in humans are called infectious agents. Parasites, fungus, viruses, and bacteria are all examples of microorganisms. Direct touch, droplets, airborne particles, and infected surfaces and objects are all potential vectors for their spread. Examples of infectious agents include the bacteria Staphylococcus aureus and the viruses Hepatitis B and Influenza A.

Infectious diseases

Infectious diseases are those caused by microorganisms and can affect people in a variety of ways. The flu, pneumonia, TB, and STDs like chlamydia and gonorrhea are just a few examples. Infections can be avoided through normal precautions, the use of personal protective gear, and careful attention to hand cleanliness.

Infection cycle/chain of infection

The transmission of an infectious disease from one host to another is described in terms of the infection cycle or chain of infection. There are a total of six components to the infection chain that must be in place. Infectious agent, reservoir, exit route, vector, entry route, susceptible host, and susceptible host. The transmission of infectious diseases can be prevented and controlled if people have a thorough understanding of these factors.

The infectious agent is the first link in the transmission chain. The bacterium or infection that triggers the illness is meant here. Bacteria, viruses, fungus, and parasites are all examples of infectious agents. The prevention and control measures necessary for one virus can be ineffective against another.

The second part is the storage facility. Infectious agents require a host organism in order to survive and spread. Humans, animals, plants, soil, water, and other natural materials all serve as reservoirs. Cholera bacteria, for instance, thrive in water that has been contaminated.

The exit door is the third component. The infectious pathogen escapes the reservoir in this way. A person's respiratory system serves as an exit point for the influenza virus.

The fourth factor is the means of communication. What this means is how the infectious agent gets from the reservoir to the host that can get sick from it. Direct touch, indirect contact, airborne transmission, droplet transmission, and vector-borne transmission are all possible ways for an infection to spread. When an infectious agent is passed from one person to another via physical contact, this is known as direct contact. Transmission of an infectious agent through an inanimate object or surface is one example of indirect contact. Transmission via droplets of respiratory secretions, such as during a cough or sneeze, is known as droplet transmission. Transmission of the infectious agent through airborne particles is known as airborne transmission. Insects like mosquitoes and ticks can act as vectors to spread disease when they bite an afflicted host.

The point of entry is the fifth component. The infectious agent enters the body through this entry point. Tetanus-causing bacteria, for instance, enter the body through open wounds or cuts.

The vulnerable host is the sixth component. This person is at risk of contracting the disease because of exposure to the infectious substance. Age, immune health, preexisting medical disorders, and genetic variables can all influence a person's susceptibility to infection.

Interrupting any one of these six steps will stop the spread of infection. Vaccination, hand hygiene, safe food handling and preparation, PPE use, and environmental controls are all viable options for achieving this goal. For effective disease control and prevention, knowledge of the transmission process is crucial.

Modes of infectious transmission

The ways in which an infection might travel from one individual to another, or from a source to a host, are known as "modes of infectious transmission." To stop the spread of infectious diseases, knowing their various ways of transmission is crucial.

Infectious diseases can spread in a number of ways, including:

Direct contact

Transmission of the disease occurs when an individual who is affected comes into contact with another individual, hence facilitating the spread of the pathogen. Sexual contact, kissing, and other forms of physical interaction are examples.

Indirect contact

Contact with an infected object or surface is the mechanism behind this type of transmission. Interacting with an infected person, for as via touching a contaminated doorknob or exchanging cutlery.

Droplet transmission

Droplets containing the infectious agent are released when an infected individual coughs, sneezes, or speaks. People who inhale or come into contact with the droplets or come into contact with the infected person are at risk of infection.

Airborne transmission

When an infectious agent is dispersed through the air and inhaled by others, this is the result. Diseases like tuberculosis, measles, and chicken pox are just a few examples.

Vector-borne transmission

In this case, the infectious agent is carried and spread by an animal or insect. Mosquitoes and ticks, respectively, are responsible for the transmission of malaria and Lyme disease.

Foodborne transmission

This happens when people consume food or drink that contains a pathogen. Salmonella, E. coli, and the norovirus are just a few examples.

Fomite transmission

This is what happens when a human becomes sick after touching a contaminated inanimate object, like a doorknob or a table.

Understanding the many routes of transmission and implementing countermeasures is crucial for limiting infectious illnesses. Preventive measures encompass several tactics, such as regular hand hygiene through the utilization of soap and water, the application of hand sanitizers, the adoption of mask-wearing practices, the observance of proper coughing and sneezing etiquette by covering the mouth and nose, and the avoidance of close contact with those exhibiting signs of illness. To stop the transmission of disease in hospitals and clinics, extra precautions are taken, such as the use of gloves and gowns, the isolation of sick patients, and the sterilization of equipment.

Standard precautions and exposure control

The healthcare industry relies heavily on standard precautions and exposure management to limit the spread of infectious diseases. Blood-borne infections and other infectious agents including bacteria, viruses, and fungus can be avoided with the use of these safety measures. They were made to be administered to everyone who needs them, whether or not they had an infectious condition.

Medical personnel have a responsibility to follow standard precautions, which are a set of rules designed to limit their exposure to potentially harmful pathogens. All individuals and their bodily fluids should be treated as potentially infectious under these recommendations. Hand hygiene, protective clothing, and safe injection procedures are all examples of standard precautions. These precautions aid in limiting the spread of disease from one individual to another.

The most important thing doctors and nurses can do to stop the spread of germs is to wash their hands regularly. Before and after interaction with each patient, after taking off gloves, and after handling potentially contaminated materials, it is important to complete hand hygiene. Those working in the medical field should disinfect their hands for at least 20 seconds with soap and water or use an alcohol-based hand sanitizer.

Another crucial step healthcare workers can take to limit the spread of disease is to use personal protective equipment (PPE). Protection gear consists of things like gloves, gowns, masks, and goggles. When working in an environment where they may come into contact with infectious agents, healthcare workers should always wear the appropriate PPE. Proper use includes taking off and disposing of PPE after each use.

Safe injection procedures are crucial for stopping the spread of disease. Needles and syringes should never be reused, and instead a fresh set should be used for each injection. If possible, a single patient should use a multi-dose vial, and just one needle per patient should be placed into the vial.

When it comes to preventing the spread of disease, exposure control is just as crucial as other measures. The term "exposure control" refers to the steps taken to reduce the likelihood of an employee contracting an infectious disease while on the job. The utilization of engineering controls like ventilation systems, as well as procedures like sharps disposal, cleaning, and disinfection, are all part of this strategy.

Disposal of used sharps is an important aspect of preventing exposure. Needles and syringes should be thrown away in a puncture-proof container right after use. The container needs to be placed as close to the sharps' point of application as is practical. No medical professional should ever use their bare hands to recap a needle or handle another potentially infectious sharp.

Preventing the spread of disease also requires regular cleaning and disinfection. After each patient use, surfaces and equipment must be cleaned and disinfected. Disinfectants used in healthcare settings should be effective and used in accordance with the product's instructions.

Ventilation systems and other forms of engineering controls are crucial in stopping the spread of disease. Clean air is essential for both patients and medical staff, and ventilation systems play a key role in this regard.

When it comes to preventing the spread of disease, standard precautions and exposure control are two of the most important measures healthcare providers can take. The danger of exposure to infectious organisms can be greatly reduced if healthcare staff are well trained in and consistently apply these procedures.

Safety resources

When talking about the methods and equipment used to keep everyone in a hospital setting safe, we often use the term "safety resources." These supplies are designed to reduce the likelihood of infections, diseases, and mishaps occurring in a medical facility. Some useful tools for ensuring a secure environment include:

Personal Protective Equipment (PPE)

Personal protective equipment (PPE) consists of any garment or piece of gear worn to shield its wearer from potential harm. Gloves, gowns, masks, and respirators are all forms of personal protective equipment. In order to stop the spread of diseases and other hazards, people wear protective gear.

Engineering controls

Modifications made to the structure or workings of a healthcare institution or its machinery are known as "engineering controls," and they serve to lessen patients' vulnerability to harm. Ventilation systems that remove dangerous airborne particles are one example of engineering controls, as are hand hygiene stations located at strategic points around the building.

Management by objectives

A healthcare facility's administrative controls are the policies and procedures it puts in place to lessen patients' chances of being exposed to harmful substances or situations. Training employees, creating infection control protocols, and strictly implementing safety laws are all examples of administrative controls.

Emergency preparedness plans

In the case of an emergency, healthcare facilities must have a strategy in place to safeguard the safety of its employees and patients. Plans for emergencies should detail how people will be evacuated, how information will be shared, and what other precautions would be done.

Safety committees

Committees composed of healthcare employees, safety committees are tasked with assessing workplaces for potential safety risks and developing plans to mitigate those dangers. To improve workplace safety, committees might analyze incident reports, carry out safety inspections, and design educational initiatives.

Hazard communication programs

Hospitals and other medical facilities have hazard communication protocols in place to inform staff of any potential dangers they may face on the job. Labeling hazardous chemicals, providing safety data sheets, and offering training to personnel on how to safely handle and dispose of these products are all part of these programs.

Reporting systems

In order to ensure that accidents and near-misses are reported and addressed in a timely way, healthcare facilities must have reporting mechanisms in place. Systems for reporting events should give workers the option to submit issues anonymously and include a way to keep tabs on incidents and identify patterns over time.

The availability of adequate safety resources is fundamental to the upkeep of a risk-free and healthy healthcare setting. Implementing and adhering to safety rules, employing appropriate PPE, and reporting incidents and near-misses are all essential for a safe healthcare environment and workforce. Healthcare employees can lessen the likelihood of workplace injuries and illnesses by cooperating and making use of available safety resources.

Safety and emergency procedures

The health and safety of both patients and medical staff depends on having well-established safety and emergency protocols in place. In order to reduce the likelihood of injury and to respond appropriately in the event of an emergency, it is crucial that healthcare staff are well versed in safety regulations and emergency procedures.

Putting on protective gear is a crucial part of any safety protocol. Personal protective equipment (PPE) consists of items like gloves, masks, and gowns that are worn by healthcare professionals to prevent the spread of disease. Healthcare workers should always wear the right PPE and be familiar with its proper use and disposal.

Using sharps containers, safety needles, and safety lancets are all vital pieces of safety equipment that should never be overlooked. Needlestick injuries, as well as other sorts of injuries that might occur during medical operations, can be avoided with the use of these devices. Medical professionals should be educated on and diligently employ the usage of all available safety equipment.

Medical professionals should be knowledgeable in basic life support and cardiopulmonary resuscitation (CPR) techniques in case of an emergency. In the case of a crisis, such as a fire or natural disaster, healthcare facilities should have emergency response plans in place. Medical professionals should be conversant with these strategies and should undergo frequent emergency response training.

Doctors and nurses should know where things like fire extinguishers and medical supplies are kept in case of an emergency. The placement of emergency exits and other safety features should be clearly marked in any healthcare facility.

The policies and procedures for patient safety and incident reporting should also be known by healthcare professionals. A mechanism for reporting and investigating patient safety occurrences should be in place at all healthcare facilities. Medical professionals should be instructed in the proper reporting procedures and strongly urged to report all instances.

Healthcare workers need to be well-versed in both safety protocols and infection control practices. Hand hygiene, isolation precautions, and washing and disinfection are all examples of these measures, all of which aim to limit the transmission of infectious diseases. In order to reduce the likelihood of an illness spreading, healthcare workers should be familiar with these protocols and continuously use them.

Education of both patients and staff is crucial to effective safety and emergency planning. Patients should be informed of their responsibilities for ensuring their own safety and given resources for sharing any concerns they may have about the quality of their care. Providers in the medical field should have proper instruction in patient education and communication.

Maintaining a safe hospital environment for both patients and medical staff depends heavily on having well-established safety and emergency procedures in place. In order to respond effectively to emergencies and keep patients safe, healthcare workers should be educated on these protocols and undergo ongoing training and education.

Risk management, quality assurance, safety procedures, incident reporting/patient safety variance reporting

Critical elements of a functional healthcare system are risk management, quality assurance, safety protocols, incident reporting, and patient safety variance reporting. These measures are crucial in reducing medical mistakes that can cause harm to patients, financial losses for hospitals, and negative publicity for doctors and hospitals. Therefore, healthcare providers must be well-versed in risk management, quality assurance, safety procedures, and incident reporting to protect patients and maintain high standards of care.

The term "risk management" describes the steps used to anticipate, assess, and reduce the likelihood of unfavorable outcomes. Risk management is the process of recognizing potential threats, evaluating how likely and severe they are, and then taking action to lessen their impact or remove them altogether. Healthcare institutions can lower the possibility of adverse events by using risk management systems to identify areas of vulnerability, create preventative measures, and conduct remedial activities.

When it comes to patient care, quality assurance is the process of making sure everything is up to par. Continuous monitoring and evaluation of healthcare processes, identification of improvement opportunities, and implementation of methods to improve the quality-of-care delivery are the primary goals of quality assurance programs. Health care facilities that use quality assurance procedures report higher patient satisfaction levels and lower overall healthcare expenditures.

Preventing harm to patients and medical staff is the primary goal of all hospitals and healthcare facilities, and this is where "safety procedures" come in. Infection control, fire prevention, hazardous material management, patient identification, and fall prevention are all examples of potential safety methods. To protect both patients and themselves, healthcare workers must adhere to established safety protocols.

Adverse incidents or near-misses in healthcare settings must be documented and reported, a procedure known as "incident reporting." Healthcare facilities can lower the chance of future adverse events by taking preventative steps and enacting corrective actions that are identified through incident reporting. All occurrences involving patients should be reported immediately to a supervisor or the risk management department by healthcare workers.

Patient safety variance reporting refers to the practice of recording and communicating information on healthcare-related occurrences involving patients' safety. It's crucial for ensuring the well-being of patients and providing them with high-quality care. Reporting patient safety variances can aid hospitals in pinpointing potential points of failure, creating protective measures, and enforcing corrective procedures.

It is the responsibility of every healthcare provider to be familiar with and follow the relevant risk management, quality assurance, safety procedure, incident reporting, and patient safety deviation reporting processes. To ensure that healthcare workers recognize the significance of these processes and their role in preventing adverse outcomes, training on them should be included in both initial and ongoing education. If healthcare workers truly care about improving patient safety and the quality of care they provide, they will take part in ongoing quality assurance and improvement efforts. By adhering to these procedures, healthcare facilities may guarantee the health and well-being of their patients.

Emergency management, identification and response

Managing medical emergencies effectively is an important part of providing quality medical treatment to patients in times of crisis. The cornerstones of emergency management are detection and action. Doctors and nurses need to be able to spot the warning indications of a medical emergency and act swiftly to keep their patients from getting worse.

Acute symptoms that can't wait for treatment are used to determine whether or not a situation is an emergency. If a patient complains of chest pain and shortness of breath, for instance, it's possible that they're having a heart attack and urgent medical attention is needed. It is also an emergency if a patient is unresponsive, has difficulty breathing, is bleeding heavily, has sustained considerable head trauma, or has had other serious injuries.

Once a medical emergency has been recognized, immediate and appropriate action must be taken to treat the patient. Stabilizing the patient's condition until aid arrives may be part of emergency response procedures. This may include summoning for more personnel or specialist equipment. The emergency care team's communication with the patient and their loved ones must be straightforward and reassuring at all times.

Protocols outlining what should be done in the event of an emergency are essential in any healthcare setting. All possible emergency situations, such as cardiac arrest, severe allergic responses, and natural disasters, should be addressed in these protocols. Staff members' responsibilities, such as who makes calls for further help and who evacuates patients, should be spelled out in the protocol as well.

Healthcare providers cannot adequately respond to situations without first receiving emergency response training. Cardiopulmonary resuscitation (CPR) and other forms of basic life support, as well as advanced life support measures including drug administration and defibrillation, should be taught to all healthcare workers. Healthcare facilities should also hold frequent emergency response drills to test the knowledge and preparedness of their employees in the event of a real disaster.

Continuous assessment and enhancement are necessary for efficient emergency management. Regular assessments of emergency response methods and procedures are recommended for healthcare facilities. The results of these assessments can be used to strengthen emergency preparedness before an actual disaster strikes.

In conclusion, emergency management is a vital part of healthcare that necessitates rapid recognition and an appropriate response to guarantee patients receive the essential care in the event of an emergency. Doctors and nurses need to be able to spot the warning indications of a medical emergency and act swiftly to keep their patients from getting worse. Protocols for handling emergencies should be put in place, and personnel should be trained and evaluated on a regular basis.

Procedures/Examinations

Here, we'll go through some of the tests and processes that MAs could experience in their line of work. Preparing patients for tests, surgeries, and treatments may involve a variety of steps, such as aiding with surgical operations, collecting specimens, running diagnostic panels, and more. Medical assistants can't do their jobs well or up to their employers' standards unless they have a thorough grasp of these tests and procedures.

Get your patients ready for their upcoming tests, operations, and therapies.

A medical assistant's primary responsibility is to get patients ready for their upcoming operations. As a medical assistant, it is your responsibility to put patients at ease and answer any questions they may have before, during, and after their visit. Here are some things to keep in mind when preparing a patient for such medical procedures:

Explain the Procedure

Inform the patient of what will happen and why it must be done before beginning any test or procedure. As a result, the patient experiences less anxiety and a greater sense of calm.

Obtain Consent

Before beginning any procedure, you should get the patient's consent. The patient must be informed of the procedure's potential side effects, benefits, and alternatives.

Check for Allergies

In order to ensure that the patient does not have an adverse reaction to any of the medications or other compounds that will be used during the treatment, it is crucial to do an allergy test beforehand.

Provide Instructions

Give the patient detailed information on how to get ready for the surgery or assessment, including whether or not they should fast, drink, or take any medications.

Assist with Preparation

The medical assistant may need to help the patient get ready for the procedure by doing things like getting them into a gown and showing them where to stand throughout the exam.

Monitor Vital Signs

Vital signs should be monitored throughout the procedure or examination, and the physician should be notified of any changes.

Offer Support

Supporting and reassuring the patient, as well as informing them of what is happening and what to expect, is crucial during the process.

Provide Post-Procedure Instructions

After the procedure, make sure the patient understands how to take any prescribed drugs, what to avoid doing, and what symptoms to look out for.

Document the Procedure

Accurate records are crucial for patient treatment and compliance with regulatory requirements. Include the date, time, provider's name, and any pertinent observations or discoveries in your documentation of the procedure.

An essential component of a medical assistant's job is getting patients ready for their upcoming exams, surgeries, and treatments. Maintain open lines of communication with the patient, get their agreement, keep an eye on their vitals, and encourage them as much as possible during the process. Accurate documentation is also crucial for patient care and for safeguarding one's legal position.

Supplies, equipment, techniques and patient instruction

Preparation for an evaluation, procedure, or therapy always includes gathering the necessary supplies and equipment. The success, safety, and efficiency of any examination or procedure performed by a medical professional depend on their having taken the time to properly prepare for it. The healthcare professional bears the responsibility of ensuring the presence and operational effectiveness of all essential supplies and equipment prior to any examination or procedure. Among these duties is making sure the materials in the examination room are stocked and in working order and making sure the treatment space is set up properly.

Various processes and tests call for an array of tools and materials. Instruments, sterile gloves, and drapes may be needed for a surgical procedure, whereas a blood pressure cuff, stethoscope, thermometer, and scale may be needed for a normal medical check. Supplies and tools are more likely to be put to their intended use if they are clearly labeled and identifiable.

Exam and procedure techniques also differ based on the nature of the treatment and individual patient requirements. Providers of medical treatment must be knowledgeable of the procedures they do and flexible enough to meet the demands of each particular patient. To achieve these goals, it is important to position the patient correctly, use the right amount of pressure, and be gentle.

To ensure the patient is ready for the examination, procedure, or therapy, it is crucial to provide them with the appropriate patient instruction. Patients should be given clear instructions on what to anticipate, how to be ready, and what they can do to have a positive and productive experience. Any pertinent information, such as fasting, hydration, medication limits, etc. The patient's trust and confidence can be bolstered, and their worries about the operation can be eased, by open and honest communication.

Getting a patient ready for a test, procedure, or treatment entails a number of steps, including making sure you have the right tools and supplies, employing the right methods for the job, and giving the patient thorough, understandable instructions. The examination or operation will be more comfortable for the patient and more successful for the healthcare professional if they have taken the time to properly prepare for it.

Surgical assisting

A medical assistant's clinical competence is incomplete without training and experience in surgical assistance. Preparing patients for surgery and assisting the surgeon during operations are common duties for medical assistants. This calls for familiarity with surgical methods and equipment, as well as an awareness of the importance of maintaining a sterile operating room.

A medical assistant's duties in the operating room include putting up the surgical table, lights, and other equipment, as well as cleaning and sterilizing the equipment and instruments that will be used during the procedure. They also help the patient get ready for surgery, which may include things like shaving and cleaning the incision.

A medical assistant's role is to aid the surgeon during surgery by doing tasks such as handing tools, keeping the operating room clean, and checking on the patient's vitals. Suturing and closing wounds may also be performed with their help.

Strong communication and interpersonal skills are just as important as technical competence in the field of surgical assisting. A medical assistant's skills in communication, anticipating the surgeon's demands, and providing emotional support to patients are all essential.

Medical assistants should have a broad understanding of both common surgical procedures and the more specialized ones. A medical assistant may help out during any number of typical surgical operations, including:

Appendectomy

In situations of appendicitis, this surgical procedure is used to remove the appendix.

Cholecystectomy

The gallbladder is removed surgically, typically because of gallstones.

Hysterectomy

This refers to the removal of a woman's uterus through surgery, which may be necessary due to cancer or other medical issues.

Mastectomy

In situations of breast cancer, this procedure entails the surgical removal of one or both breasts.

Tonsillectomy

In cases of chronic tonsillitis, tonsillectomy surgery is performed to remove the tonsils.

Medical assistants may be required to provide care for patients both before and after surgical procedures. Some examples of this type of post-operative care are taking vital signs, giving medication, and instructing the patient on how to care for a wound.

Medical assistants might specialize in surgical support by gaining further education or certification. The Certified Clinical Medical Assistant (CCMA) credential is available through the National Healthcareer Association, and it features a surgical assisting curriculum. Further, one can become a Certified Surgical Technologist (CST) by completing a surgical technology program and passing an exam administered by the National Board of Surgical Technology and Surgical Assisting. Although certification is not essential to work as a surgical assistant, having it can show employers that you're dedicated to your field's advancement.

A medical assistant's competence in surgical assistance is essential. Strong communication and interpersonal skills are essential, as well as technical knowledge of surgical processes and instruments. If a medical assistant is considering a career change, they might want to look into surgical assisting programs.

Specimen collection techniques

Collection and processing of biological fluids and tissues for laboratory analysis is known as specimen collection. It plays a major role in both medical diagnosis and patient treatment. Reliable test results and better patient outcomes depend on the proper collection and treatment of specimens. Various methods of collecting specimens and their significance in medical diagnosis will be covered in this article.

Blood Collection

One of the most popular forms of specimen collection is blood samples. The median cubital vein in the antecubital fossa, the cephalic vein, and the basilic vein are the most often used veins for blood collection. There are a variety of collection tubes available for blood that can be used for various diagnostic procedures. Serum separator tubes, used for chemistry testing, heparin tubes, used for various chemistry and coagulation studies, and EDTA tubes, used for hematology tests, are all common types of blood collection tubes. Patient identification information such as name, DOB, and medical record number should be clearly printed on the label of each blood collection tube.

Urinalysis

The term "urinalysis" refers to the process of collecting and analyzing urine for diagnostic purposes. To prevent contamination from the genital area, a clean-catch midstream specimen is often taken. The patient should wash their genitalia before providing a urine sample, and the first urine should be thrown away. A sterile container bearing the patient's name and identification should be used for collection.

Stool Collection

Intestinal disorders, such as infection or inflammation, can be diagnosed through stool collection. Using a sterile swab or other collection instrument, a small sample of stool is taken. In order to enhance the likelihood of finding any pathogens, the samples should be obtained from several parts of the feces. A sterile container bearing the patient's name should be used for the specimen.

Sputum Collection

Collecting sputum is a common diagnostic procedure for respiratory diseases like malignancy and infection. Aseptic containers are employed for the purpose of gathering expectorated respiratory secretions subsequent to the patient being instructed to engage in forceful coughing. Avoiding contamination requires collecting the samples first thing in the morning, before the patient has had anything to eat or drink. Patient information should be included on the label attached to the specimen.

Cerebrospinal Fluid (CSF) Collection

Cerebrospinal fluid (CSF) is the fluid that bathes the brain and spinal cord. Meningitis and encephalitis can be diagnosed with a cerebrospinal fluid (CSF) collection. After placing the patient in the fetal position, the lower back is often cleaned with an antiseptic solution. The fluid is extracted by inserting a needle into the spinal canal. A sterile container bearing the patient's name and identification should be used for collection.

Tissue Biopsy

Collecting a sample of tissue, called a "biopsy," allows for closer inspection of the affected area. Different techniques are used to take biopsies from various parts of the body. A liver biopsy requires inserting a needle into the liver to retrieve a sample, while a skin biopsy requires removing a small piece of skin. A sterile container bearing the patient's name should be used for the specimen.

The methods used to collect specimens are pivotal in-patient care and diagnosis. Accurate test results and improved patient outcomes can be achieved by careful collection and storage of specimens. To protect the safety of patients and healthcare workers, clinicians should be familiar with the various collecting methods and adhere to established guidelines.

Laboratory panels and selected tests

When it comes to diagnosing and treating illnesses, laboratory testing is crucial. To aid in the diagnosis and treatment of medical disorders, medical laboratory technicians and technologists undertake a wide range of laboratory tests and analysis. Here we'll go through some of the most often prescribed laboratory tests and panel analyses by doctors.

Complete Blood Count (CBC)

The red blood cell count, white blood cell count, and platelet count are all measured in a complete blood count (CBC) blood test. This analysis has the potential to detect a wide range of illnesses, including blood abnormalities, infections, and more.

Basic Metabolic Panel (BMP)

Electrolyte levels, blood sugar levels, and renal function can all be determined with a BMP. Electrolytes, which are found in the blood, are minerals that aid in the regulation of many body activities, particularly those of the muscles and nerves. Patients experiencing symptoms including weakness, weariness, or confusion may require this test to monitor the efficacy of their drugs or for diagnostic purposes.

Comprehensive Metabolic Panel (CMP)

Electrolytes, hyperglycemia, kidney and liver function can all be determined with the help of a CMP blood test. Liver disease, kidney disease, and diabetes are just some of the illnesses that can be detected and monitored using this test.

Lipid Panel

Cholesterol and triglyceride levels can be determined using a blood test called a "lipid panel." Elevated blood levels of cholesterol and triglycerides have been found to be correlated with an increased susceptibility to cardiovascular disease and stroke. The risk of cardiovascular disease is commonly evaluated with this test.

Thyroid Function Panel

Thyroid hormone and thyroid stimulating hormone (TSH) levels can be determined with a blood test called a thyroid function panel. Thyroid hormones play a role in controlling thermoregulation, heart rate, and metabolism. Patients experiencing symptoms like weariness, weight gain, or hair loss are frequently sent for this test.

Urinalysis

A urinalysis can detect things such as proteins, carbohydrates, and red blood cells in the urine. Kidney problems, urinary tract infections, and even diabetes can all be detected and monitored with this simple test.

Stool Analysis

Stool analysis is a test used to detect bacteria, parasites, and other contaminants in human waste. Conditions including inflammatory bowel disease and gastrointestinal infections can be diagnosed using this test.

Microbiology Culture

Microbiology cultures are used to detect the presence of microorganisms like bacteria and fungi in samples of bodily fluids, tissues, and other things. This test can aid in the diagnosis of infections and the selection of appropriate treatments.

Other specialist tests may be ordered by doctors after considering a patient's symptoms, medical history, and physical exam results. Accurate and trustworthy results can only be achieved by strict adherence to established laboratory processes and quality control measures by medical laboratory technicians and technologists. In addition to using PPE and keeping a clean and organized workplace, these measures should be taken to limit the transmission of disease.

Overview of Body Systems and Their Functions

The human body is an intricate network of specialized organs that work together. Different systems serve different purposes and have different organizational frameworks, yet they all contribute to an organism's health and survival. Healthcare providers cannot adequately serve their patients without a deep familiarity with the human body and its many complex processes. The cardiovascular, digestive, endocrine, cutaneous, lymphatic, muscular, neurological, reproductive, respiratory, skeletal, and sensory systems will all get some attention here.

The organs, tissues, and cells that make up each system will be discussed, as will their respective roles and interactions within the body. We'll also take a look at how these various systems interact with one another to keep the body in a steady state of balance, or homeostasis.

In order to provide the best care for their patients, medical practitioners need a thorough understanding of the human body and its systems, including its functioning and interconnections.

Anatomy of the circulatory system

The cardiovascular system, or circulatory system, is in charge of pumping blood throughout the body to supply cells with oxygen and nutrition and remove waste. The circulatory system includes the heart, the arteries, and the blood. A healthcare provider's ability to recognize and diagnose circulatory system issues hinges on his or her familiarity of the system's anatomy.

The cardiac muscle is found in the chest, between the lungs. Its primary function is to transport blood to all parts of the body. The atria are the upper two chambers of the heart, whereas the ventricles are the lower two chambers. The right atrium receives deoxygenated blood from the body, which is subsequently pushed into the right ventricle. The blood is propelled by the right ventricle towards the lungs in order to undergo oxygenation. The left atrium of the heart receives oxygenated blood and subsequently transports it to the left ventricle. The aorta is responsible for transporting oxygenated blood to the rest of the body after it has been pumped by the left ventricle.

The circulatory system would be incomplete without the blood vessels. The human circulatory system consists of a complex arrangement of arteries, veins, and capillaries. Arteries play a vital role in the distribution of oxygenated blood from the heart to different tissues and organs in the body, while veins assist the circulation of deoxygenated blood back to the heart. Capillaries, the smallest blood veins, play a crucial role in delivering oxygen and nutrients to the cells of the body.

The final part of the circulatory system is blood. The components of whole blood are plasma, RBCs, WBCs, and platelets. Yellowish plasma contains water, electrolytes, and proteins; it accounts for around 55% of blood. Erythrocytes, also known as red blood cells, transport oxygen from the lungs to the rest of the body's tissues. Leukocytes, also known as white blood cells, protect the body from pathogens and other harmful substances. Platelets are a type of blood cell that helps stop bleeding by clumping together to create clots.

The circulatory system is a sophisticated network that removes waste and transports oxygen and nutrients to the body's cells. The heart, the vascular system, and the blood all play a significant role in the body's ability to pump blood efficiently to all parts. For accurate diagnosis and treatment of circulatory issues, medical personnel require in-depth knowledge of cardiovascular anatomy.

Physiology of the circulatory system

The cardiovascular system, or circulatory system, is in charge of distributing blood, blood cells, oxygen, minerals, hormones, and waste products throughout the body. The cardiovascular system includes the heart, the aorta, the veins, and the capillaries, as well as the blood itself. Maintaining homeostasis and satisfying the metabolic demands of the body require the coordinated action of these components, which is what the physiology of the circulatory system is all about.

Heart Physiology

The heart is a muscle that circulates blood throughout the body. The right atrium, right ventricle, left atrium, and left ventricle make up its four chambers. The right atrium receives blood from the body before it is pumped by the right ventricle to the lungs. The left atrium receives oxygenated blood from the body, while the left ventricle pumps the blood to the rest of the body.

Electrical signals regulate muscle contraction and relaxation in the heart. The sinoatrial (SA) node in the right atrium functions as the heart's intrinsic pacemaker. It produces electrical impulses that go throughout the atrium and squeeze it shut. A minor delay is introduced at the atrioventricular (AV) node so that the ventricles can fill with blood before contracting.

Blood Vessels Physiology

The function of blood vessels is to transport blood to all parts of the body. Blood that has been oxygenated by the heart is transported by arteries, whereas blood that has been depleted of oxygen is returned to the heart via veins. Capillaries are the thin-walled, small blood vessels that link arteries to veins and facilitate the transport of oxygen, nutrients, and waste products from the blood to the tissues.

The walls of arteries are quite muscular and can contract and relax to control blood flow. Arterial walls are smooth on the inside, which helps keep blood from clotting. Veins' thin walls allow the surrounding tissues' muscular contractions to propel blood back toward the heart. In addition, they feature one-way valves that stop blood from reversing direction.

Physiology of Blood

Blood is a unique bodily fluid because it carries oxygen, nutrients, hormones, and metabolites to all parts of the body. It consists of plasma, RBCs, WBCs, and PLTs (platelet-rich plasma).

About 55% of the total volume of blood is plasma, the blood's liquid component. There are electrolytes, proteins, and hormones in there as well. Oxygen is transported throughout the body by red blood cells (RBCs), which originate in the lungs. Hemoglobin, an oxygen-binding protein, is found in red blood cells. WBCs, or white blood cells, are an important aspect of the immune system. Platelets assist stop bleeding by forming clots in the blood.

Regulation of Blood Pressure

What we mean when we talk about "blood pressure" is the pressure that the blood is putting on the artery walls. The heart, blood vessels, and nerve system all work together in intricate ways to control it. A pressure wave is created by the heart's contraction and moves through the arterial system. Systolic blood pressure refers to this measurement. Arterial pressure drops when the heart slows down its beating. The diastolic reading is the one that matters.

Age, sex, genetics, nutrition, exercise, and stress all play a role in determining blood pressure. High blood pressure, often known as hypertension, is a common medical disease that can have dire consequences if left untreated. Medications and behavioral modification are common treatments.

Oxygen, nutrition, hormones, and waste products are all transported throughout the body through the circulatory system, which is a complicated network in and of itself. The heart, blood vessels, and blood must all work together for it to be effective.

Functions of blood

Blood is classified as a form of connective tissue that circulates throughout the entirety of the human body, facilitating the transportation of vital substances such as oxygen and nutrients to cells and organs, while concurrently eliminating waste products for subsequent disposal. Blood is composed of four primary constituents, namely plasma, platelets, white blood cells, and red blood cells. All of these chemicals play a crucial role in facilitating the optimal operation of the circulatory system.

Erythrocytes, commonly referred to as red blood cells, constitute the predominant cell type inside the blood. Erythrocytes transport oxygen from the pulmonary system to various organs and tissues inside the body. Hemoglobin, a protein present in red blood cells (RBCs), serves the function of facilitating the transportation of oxygen from the lungs to various tissues and organs throughout the body. Carbon dioxide is generated as a byproduct of cellular respiration and subsequently conveyed by erythrocytes to the pulmonary system for elimination.

Leukocytes, or white blood cells, are essential to the body's immune response. They protect the body from germs and viruses and dispose of damaged or dead cells. distinct types of white blood cells have distinct purposes. Antigen-recognizing cells such as neutrophils and antibody-secreting lymphocytes are among the first to respond to an infection.

Platelets, sometimes called thrombocytes, are tiny cells that help the blood clot. They coagulate into a plug that seals off the broken blood artery. During the clotting process, platelets secrete substances that stimulate many other cells.

About 55% of the volume of blood is plasma, the blood's liquid component. It is mostly water, however it does have certain proteins like albumin, globulins, and fibrinogen in it. Plasma helps control body temperature and transports nutrients, hormones, and waste products throughout the body.

Overall, blood is crucial to the body's ability to maintain homeostasis, serving a wide variety of roles. Some examples of these roles are:

Transportation

Oxygen, nutrients, and hormones are delivered to cells by the blood, and waste products like carbon dioxide and lactic acid are removed.

Regulation

The body's temperature, acid-base balance, and fluid levels are all maintained by blood.

Protection

Blood contains both white blood cells, which help fight off illnesses and foreign invaders, and platelets, which help stop bleeding.

Homeostasis

The body's internal environment relies on blood to help keep things like temperature, pH, and fluid balance steady.

Blood plays an essential role in homeostasis and health maintenance. Understanding the physiology of the circulatory system is crucial for providing good patient care, and each component of blood plays a specific role in these processes.

Digestive system anatomy

In order for the body to absorb and use nutrients from food, the digestive system must first break them down into smaller molecules. It's a sophisticated system that depends on a number of organs, all of which perform unique tasks.

Mechanical breakdown occurs in the teeth, and chemical breakdown occurs thanks to enzymes in saliva, marking the beginning of the digestive process. Next, the food enters the stomach, where acid and digestive enzymes finish the job of breaking it down.

The small intestine receives the food that has been partially digested from the stomach. Villi and microvilli are anatomical structures characterized by finger-like projections that form a lining along the surface of the small intestine. These structures serve to augment the overall surface area of the small intestine, hence facilitating more efficient absorption of nutrients.

Water and electrolytes from the undigested food are absorbed by the large intestine (or colon), which is also responsible for generating excrement. The excretion of excrement occurs through the rectum and anus.

Several auxiliary organs in the digestive tract also play a role in breaking down food. The pancreas, liver, and gallbladder all fall within this category. Bile is synthesized within the hepatic organ and has a crucial role in facilitating the breakdown and absorption of lipids within the gastrointestinal tract, particularly in the small intestine. Bile is discharged from the gallbladder into the small intestine as required. The pancreas releases digestive enzymes into the small intestine, facilitating the breakdown of carbohydrates, proteins, and fats during the process of digestion.

The digestive system is essential for keeping the body's energy and nutrient levels stable. The digestive system's efficiency has far-reaching implications for one's health and well-being.

Physiology of the digestive system

The digestive system is in charge of separating nutrients from meals into smaller pieces that the body can use. The process of food digestion, involving both mechanical and chemical mechanisms, initiates in the oral cavity, progresses within the gastric region, and culminates in the small intestine, which serves as the primary site for nutrient absorption.

In the mouth, food is broken down mechanically by the teeth and tongue and mixed with saliva. Amylase is an enzyme found in saliva that catalyzes the first step in the chemical breakdown of carbohydrates. After being broken down into smaller pieces and combined with saliva, food is shaped into a bolus and swallowed.

Muscular contractions in the stomach aid in the mechanical digestion of food, while hydrochloric acid and enzymes like pepsin aid in the chemical digestion. Proteins are digested and dangerous germs are killed by the stomach's acidic environment. This amalgam is known as chyme, and it is gradually secreted into the villi of the small intestine.

The majority of nutritional absorption occurs within the small intestine. Small intestinal villi and microvilli are finger-like projections that increase absorption area by spreading out across the intestinal wall. Enzymes created by the pancreas and small intestine break down nutrients like proteins, lipids, and carbs. After being ingested, these nutrients make their way to the liver for digestion.

Solid feces are formed when the large intestine (colon) extracts water and electrolytes from the undigested meal. The feces are passed out of the body via the rectum and the anus.

Hormones and nervous system pathways coordinate digestive function. Food triggers the release of hormones such gastrin and secretin, which in turn increase digestive enzyme production and digestive motility. Digestive function is also regulated by the neurological system, with the parasympathetic nervous system aiding digestion and the sympathetic nervous system suppressing it.

Getting the nutrients, the body requires from food is mostly dependent on the digestive system. Multiple diseases and disorders, including malabsorption syndromes, inflammatory bowel disease, and gastrointestinal malignancies, can result from digestive system dysfunction.

The Endocrine System: Anatomy

The endocrine system comprises a complex network of glands and organs that are responsible for the secretion of hormones, hence regulating several physiological processes within the human body. The endocrine system comprises various glands, including the pituitary gland, thyroid gland, adrenal glands, pancreas, ovaries (in females), and testes (in males). The coordination of these organs is essential for regulating various physiological processes including as development, metabolism, and reproduction.

At the back of the brain is the pituitary gland, also called the "master gland," which is in charge of producing and secreting a number of hormones that regulate the functioning of the body's other endocrine glands. Thyroid-stimulating hormone (TSH), secreted by the pituitary gland, controls the production of thyroid hormones, which in turn affect the body's metabolic rate. The pituitary gland is responsible for producing growth hormone, a hormone that controls skeletal and muscular growth from childhood into adulthood.

Hormones produced by the thyroid gland in the neck control metabolic rate, heart rate, and core body temperature. Thyroxine (T4) and triiodothyronine (T3) are the two main hormones secreted by the thyroid gland, and they regulate the pace at which the body utilizes energy. Hormone synthesis by the thyroid gland is controlled by TSH, which is secreted by the pituitary gland.

The hormones produced by the adrenal glands, which sit on top of the kidneys, control the body's response to stress, blood pressure, and electrolyte balance. Cortisol, produced by the adrenal gland, controls the body's reaction to stress and inflammation. Aldosterone, produced by the adrenal gland, controls the amount of sodium and potassium in the blood.

Behind the stomach is an organ called the pancreas, which secretes hormones that control blood sugar. Insulin is secreted by the pancreas and reduces blood sugar by increasing the efficiency with which cells take up glucose. Glucagon is produced by the pancreas and causes the liver to release glucose into the bloodstream, hence increasing blood sugar levels.

The ovaries secrete hormones that control the female reproductive system, including the monthly cycle, fertility, and pregnancy. The ovaries play a crucial role in the preparation of the uterus for potential pregnancy and in the regulation of growth and development of the female reproductive system through the secretion of the hormones estrogen and progesterone.

Testosterone is a hormone produced by the testes in men that controls the growth of primary sex traits like facial and body hair, as well as secondary sex characteristics like the size and shape of the testes.

The endocrine system is vitally important since it controls many different bodily functions. Diabetes, thyroid problems, and infertility are just some of the conditions that can result from malfunctions in the endocrine system.

Anatomy of the skin

The skin is the biggest organ and acts as a protective barrier between the inside of the body and the outside. It's crucial for maintaining a healthy internal climate, warding off infections and injuries, and allowing for the reception of sensory information. There are three basic parts to the skin: the epidermis, the dermis, and the subcutaneous tissue.

There are four or five layers in the epidermis, the outermost layer of skin, depending on where you are. Keratinocytes are the cells responsible for making the protein keratin, which gives skin its strength and ability to repel water. Melanocytes can be found in the epidermis, and they are responsible for producing the pigment melanin that gives skin its color and protects it from UV radiation.

The dermis is the skin's middle layer and is home to several tissues and organs like blood vessels, nerves, and connective tissue. It contains fibers of collagen and elastin, which give the skin its suppleness and resilience, and serves as the skin's structural support system. The sebaceous glands, sweat glands, and hair follicles are all found in the dermis.

Fat cells predominate in the subcutaneous tissue, also called the hypodermis, which is the deepest layer of skin. It serves as a source of insulation and padding for the body in addition to a reservoir for energy.

A number of specialized cells and structures, essential to immunological function and sensory perception, are located in the skin. There are several different types of sensory cells: Merkel cells, which are involved in touch sense, Langerhans cells, which help identify and respond to infections, and Meissner's corpuscles and Pacinian corpuscles are sensory receptors that are responsible for detecting light touch and vibration, respectively.

There are many different layers and structures that make up the skin, and they all contribute to keeping this organ healthy and functioning properly.

Physiology of the skin

The biggest organ in the human body is the skin. This organ has many important functions, including acting as a barrier against harmful environmental factors, controlling core body temperature, and regulating fluid and electrolyte levels. Sensation, thermoregulation, protection, and metabolic processes are only few of the many functions of the skin's intricate physiology. In this post, we'll look at the skin's many roles and how they affect an individual's health and happiness.

Protection

The skin's primary role is to defend the body against environmental hazards such harmful chemicals and pathogens. The skin functions as a protective barrier, keeping harmful bacteria and chemicals out of the body. The epidermis is the outermost layer of skin, and it is made up of several layers of keratinized cells that work together to create a barrier that is both waterproof and impermeable. Langerhans cells are found in the epidermis and aid in the detection and elimination of potentially harmful organisms.

Sensation

Touch, pressure, temperature, and pain are only few of the sensations detected and sent to the brain via the skin. Numerous sensory receptors, each sensitive to a somewhat different set of stimuli, are found in the skin. Light touch is sensed by Meissner's corpuscles, while deep pressure and vibration are picked up by Pacinian corpuscles. The sensory function of the skin aids in communication with and protection against the surrounding environment.

Thermoregulation

The skin also plays a vital role in maintaining a comfortable internal temperature. The skin's enormous network of blood vessels can either assist cool the body down or keep it warm. The skin's blood vessels widen in response to a high ambient temperature, bringing more blood to the surface and facilitating heat loss by radiation and convection. The skin's blood vessels, on the other hand, narrow when the body senses a drop in temperature, resulting in less blood being pumped to the surface while the core temperature remains same.

Metabolism

The skin plays a role in a number of important metabolic processes that contribute to the maintenance of the body as a whole. Vitamin D, an essential component for calcium homeostasis, bone health, and immunological function, is synthesized by the skin when exposed to sunlight. Additionally, the skin produces sebum, a lipid-rich material that serves to both keep the skin supple and prevent microbial and fungal diseases.

The skin's complex physiology allows it to serve many vital roles in maintaining the body's health. Protecting your skin from the elements, drinking plenty of water, and living a healthy lifestyle that includes eating right and getting regular exercise are all essential for keeping your skin in good condition. If you develop a rash, discoloration, or lesion, or otherwise notice a change in the appearance or texture of your skin, you should visit a doctor. Preventing further damage and improving overall skin health is possible through early detection and treatment of skin disorders.

Lymphatic system anatomy

The lymphatic system is an intricate network of veins, lymph nodes, organs, and tissues that aids in the body's immune response and regulates fluid levels. The lymphatic system cooperates closely with the circulatory system to drain interstitial fluid, proteins, and waste from tissues back into the blood. This page provides an in-depth look at the lymphatic system's anatomy.

You can think of the lymphatic system as having three primary parts:

The lymphatic system's vessels

Lymphatic vessels are tubular structures with narrow walls that carry lymph fluid. Lymphatic vessels resemble blood vessels structurally but have thinner walls and more valves to prevent lymph from flowing in the wrong direction. Lymphatic vessels are able to take in interstitial fluid, proteins, and waste materials from tissues because they are more porous than blood vessels.

Lymph nodes

To eliminate harmful items like germs, viruses, and cancer cells from the lymph fluid, the body contains tiny, bean-shaped structures called lymph nodes. Lymphocytes, which are found in the lymph nodes, are specialized immune cells that aid in the body's immune response to foreign invaders.

Lymphoid organs

The thymus, spleen, tonsils, adenoids, and Peyer's patches in the small intestine are all examples of lymphoid organs. Lymphoid organs are vital to immune defense because of the large number of lymphocytes and other immune cells they house.

The lymphatic vessels develop from the tiny capillaries that are scattered throughout the tissues. These capillaries are specialized to remove fluid, proteins, and waste from surrounding tissues. Larger lymphatic veins form when lymphatic capillaries join together; these carry lymph fluid to the lymph nodes. Lymph nodes are specialized organs that filter lymph fluid and rid the body of harmful bacteria and viruses.

When lymph fluid leaves a lymph node, it travels via bigger lymphatic channels before returning to the circulatory system via the thoracic duct, which empties into the left subclavian vein.

Lymphatic system physiology

The lymphatic system is an intricate network of organs, tissues, blood arteries, and fluid that helps the body's immune system work properly and keeps its fluid levels stable. Lymph, a transparent fluid containing immune cells and waste materials, is filtered and transported throughout the body through lymphatic veins and lymph nodes. The process by which fats are taken up and conveyed from the gastrointestinal tract to the circulatory system is facilitated by the lymphatic system. This chapter will extensively examine the role and functionality of the lymphatic system.

The lymphatic system is responsible for a number of crucial bodily processes, including:

Maintaining immune function

Lymphatic fluid contains immune cells that aid in the body's defense against infection and disease, making the lymphatic system an essential component of the immune system. The lymph nodes are the immune system's filtering system, eliminating harmful substances and debris.

The lymphatic system is also crucial in the process of absorbing and transporting fats from the digestive tract to the circulatory system. The lipids we eat are absorbed by lymphatic veins in the small intestine called lacteals, which then carry them to the circulation via the thoracic duct.

Maintaining fluid balance

The lymphatic system is responsible for returning surplus fluid from the tissues to the bloodstream, so assisting the circulatory system in keeping the body's fluid levels stable. This aids in the avoidance of edema and swelling.

Removing waste products

The lymphatic system aids in the elimination of metabolic byproducts, such as excess fluid, cellular waste, and immune system detritus.

Muscular System Anatomy

The muscles are an intricate system of organs and tissues that help the body move and keep it stable. The force necessary for motion is generated by contractile structures called muscles. In addition to supporting the body's structure, they produce body heat and move vital organs like the heart and intestines.

There are three major forms of muscle tissue in the body, and they are referred to as skeletal, smooth, and cardiac. These several muscle groups all serve different purposes and display distinct anatomical properties.

Connected to the skeleton, skeletal muscles allow for free movement. Muscle fibers are long, cylindrical cells that make up the muscle. Many nuclei are packed into these threads, and their alternating light and dark bands give them a striated appearance. Conscious control and quick, powerful contractions of skeletal muscle tissue are possible.

The walls of hollow organs including the blood arteries, stomach, and intestines are made of smooth muscle tissue. The cells that make up this structure are shorter and spindle-shaped; they lack striae and have a single nucleus. Involuntary means not under voluntary control; this describes smooth muscular tissue well. Compared to skeletal muscle, cardiac muscle contracts more slowly and weakly, but it may stay contracted for much longer.

The only place you'll find cardiac muscle is in your heart. The striations and numerous nuclei give it a look not dissimilar to that of skeletal muscle. Like smooth muscle tissue, however, this one is involuntary. The heart's muscle tissue constantly contracts in a rhythmic pattern to circulate blood.

Muscle function depends on a number of structures beyond the muscle tissue itself. Muscles adhere to bones via tendons, which are stiff, fibrous connective structures. Muscle contractions generate force, and these fibers carry that force to the joints to cause motion. Ligaments are connective tissues that attach bones to other bones and resemble tendons in structure. They help keep joints in place and stop unnecessary wiggles.

The nervous system plays a vital role in the regulation of skeletal muscle. Muscle contractions are initiated through the transmission of neural signals from the central nervous system, comprising the brain and spinal cord, to specialized motor neurons.

Muscles can only do their job if they receive enough oxygenated blood. A system of capillaries carries oxygenated blood to each muscle fiber in the body. Muscles rely on these capillaries for oxygen, nutrition, and waste removal (carbon dioxide).

The musculoskeletal system plays a crucial role in movement and general bodily function. To coordinate and regulate movement and to maintain homeostasis in the body, it works closely with other systems like the neurological, cardiovascular, and respiratory ones. Maintaining healthy and functional muscles throughout life requires a balanced diet, regular exercise, and enough of rest.

Skeletal muscle physiology

Muscles in the skeleton allow humans to walk and stand upright. The ability to walk, run, and jump is made possible by these muscles, which are under the guidance of the brain. Muscle contraction and relaxation are facilitated by a number of physiological mechanisms unique to skeletal muscles. Medical personnel need an understanding of skeletal muscle physiology in order to properly diagnose and treat muscular problems.

Muscle fibers in skeletal muscles are organized into myofibrils. Myofibrils are the structural units of striated muscles, and they house the contractile proteins known as sarcomeres. Skeletal muscles contain both fast-twitch (Type II) and slow-twitch (Type I) fibers.

Smaller in size, slow-twitch fibers rely on oxygen-rich blood for their energy production and have a high oxidative metabolic capability. These muscles are primarily used in endurance sports like long-distance running because of their incredible resistance to fatigue. However, fast-twitch fibers, which use anaerobic metabolism, are bigger in diameter. Highly fatigable, they are best reserved for sports like sprinting and weightlifting that call for brief periods of maximum effort.

In order for skeletal muscles to contract, a nerve impulse must first travel to them from a motor neuron. The neurotransmitter acetylcholine is secreted by motor neurons; it binds to receptors on muscle fibers, whereupon calcium ions are released from the sarcoplasmic reticulum. Troponin is a protein that undergoes a conformational shift when calcium ions connect to it. This change makes the protein's binding sites for myosin, a thick filament in the sarcomere, accessible.

Once bound, myosin forms cross-bridges with actin, another thin filament in the sarcomere. By drawing the thin filaments into the center of the sarcomere, myosin utilises the energy created from hydrolyzing ATP to contract the muscle. If there are calcium ions in the sarcoplasm and ATP is accessible, the cross-bridge cycling mechanism will proceed.

When nerve impulses from the motor neuron stop, the skeletal muscles relax. Since calcium ions have been removed from the sarcoplasm, the release of acetylcholine has ceased. The concentration of calcium ions in the sarcoplasm is lowered as a result of active transport back into the sarcoplasmic reticulum. By resuming its native shape, troponin is able to prevent myosin from binding and release itself from actin cross-bridges. When the muscle is in rest, it lengthens back to its previous size.

The number of cross-bridges generated between myosin and actin determines the strength of skeletal muscle contraction. The number of motor units recruited, the concentration of calcium ions, and the amount of adenosine triphosphate (ATP) all play roles. When many nerve impulses are sent to the muscle in rapid succession, a process known as summation takes place, increasing the force of contraction.

Muscle contraction and relaxation are facilitated by a number of physiological mechanisms unique to skeletal muscles. Skeletal muscles contract when a nerve impulse from a motor neuron causes the sarcoplasmic reticulum to release calcium ions. Myosin binds to troponin, which opens binding sites for calcium ions. Myosin then binds to actin, creating cross-bridges that allow the muscle to contract. Stopping nerve impulses triggers skeletal muscle relaxation by actively transporting calcium ions back into the sarcoplasmic reticulum and reverting troponin to its resting state.

Physiology of smooth muscle

The walls of organs like the gastrointestinal tract, blood arteries, and urinary tract are made up of smooth muscles, which are involuntary muscles. Smooth muscles contract involuntarily in response to diverse stimuli, in contrast to skeletal muscles, which are under voluntary control. Here we'll go through the physiology of smooth muscle, covering topics like its anatomy, how it contracts, and how it's controlled.

Structure of Smooth Muscle

In contrast to striated skeletal and cardiac muscle cells, the spindle-shaped myocytes that make up smooth muscle are unpatterned. Their dimensions are 20-500 times smaller than those of skeletal muscle cells: 2-10 microns in diameter and 2-10 microns in length. There is only one nucleus in the cells that make up the walls of organs, which are made up of smooth muscle. These sheets of smooth muscle cells can synchronize their contraction and relaxation movements.

Similar to the arrangement of actin and myosin in skeletal muscle, contractile proteins are found in smooth muscle cells. However, in smooth muscle, striations are not present due to a distinct arrangement of these proteins. Both actin and myosin filaments in smooth muscle are attached to the cell membrane, while the former is linked to dense bodies found throughout the cytoplasm. Smooth muscle cells shorten during contraction because actin filaments slip across myosin filaments.

Contraction Mechanism of Smooth Muscle

Calcium ions (Ca2+) enter the cell from the surrounding fluid or the sarcoplasmic reticulum, setting off the contraction of smooth muscle. Myosin light chain kinase (MLCK) is activated when Ca2+ ions bind to the regulatory protein calmodulin in response to a stimulus such a nerve impulse or hormonal signal. Myosin light chain kinase (MLCK) phosphorylates myosin light chain, enabling actin-binding of myosin heads and contraction.

Latch state is a steady and persistent contraction unique to smooth muscle that allows the muscle to retain tension for extended periods of time with minimal energy expenditure. This is because myosin-actin cross-bridges dissociate slowly in smooth muscle.

Regulation of Smooth Muscle Contraction

Nerve impulses, hormones, and environmental factors all play roles in controlling the contraction of smooth muscle. Smooth muscle in the walls of organs like the gastrointestinal tract, respiratory system, and blood vessels are contracted by the autonomic nervous system. Smooth muscle contraction is regulated by the nervous system, with stimulation coming from the sympathetic branch and relaxation from the parasympathetic.

Hormones like adrenaline, norepinephrine, and oxytocin can either increase or decrease smooth muscle contraction. While epinephrine and norepinephrine cause vasoconstriction by stimulating the contraction of smooth muscle in blood vessels, oxytocin causes the contraction of smooth muscle in the uterus.

The contraction of smooth muscle can also be controlled by local factors such as variations in pH, oxygen, and carbon dioxide levels, and the presence of chemicals like histamine and prostaglandins.

The contraction of blood vessels, the flow of food through the digestive tract, and the contraction of the uterus during delivery are all regulated by a specific type of muscle tissue called smooth muscle. In both form and function, smooth muscle cells differ from their skeletal and cardiac counterparts. They're unstriped and controlled by nerve impulses, hormones, and even environmental cues in the immediate vicinity to maintain a gradual, constant contraction.

Functioning of the Heart's Muscles

Myocardium is another name for the specific muscular tissue that makes up the heart. Cardiac muscle is essential to the function of the heart, which is responsible for pumping blood throughout the body. This article will cover the electrical and mechanical properties of cardiac muscle in addition to its anatomical structure.

Anatomy of Cardiac Muscle:

Under a microscope, cardiac muscle cells seem striped because they are striated. They branch and intertwine to produce a network that facilitates the rapid conduction of electrical impulses throughout the heart. Intercalated discs are specialized junctions between cells that facilitate the exchange of ions through gap junctions. In doing so, an electrical syncytium is formed, allowing the heart to beat as one muscle.

Blood vessels are abundant in cardiac muscle, which is important since the heart needs oxygen and nourishment. Oxygenated blood is delivered to the heart through the coronary arteries, while deoxygenated blood is drained from the heart by the cardiac veins.

Physiology of Cardiac Muscle:

Electrical Properties

The heart muscle contracts in a coordinated and rhythmic fashion because of its special electrical characteristics. The sinoatrial (SA) node is a collection of cells in the right atrium that sends out the electrical impulse that triggers each heartbeat. After receiving the electrical signal, the atria contract and force blood into the ventricles.

The signal then travels to the heart's atrioventricular (AV) node. Because of the AV node's gatekeeping function, the ventricles have time to fill with blood before contracting. The bundle of His and Purkinje fibers carries the electrical signal from the AV node to the ventricles, where it causes the ventricles to contract in unison.

Ion transport through the cell membrane is essential for the electrical characteristics of heart muscle. In instance, calcium ion mobility is critically important in controlling muscle cell contraction. $Ca2+$ ions are released from the intracellular sarcoplasmic reticulum in response to an electrical stimulus in cardiac muscle cells. In order for the muscle cell to contract, calcium ions must first connect to a protein called troponin, setting off a cascade of chemical reactions.

Mechanical Properties

The heart's contractile muscle has special mechanical qualities that allow for quick and powerful contractions. Muscle fibers are short and branched so that more cells may communicate with one another, leading to a more powerful and coordinated contraction.

Calcium availability in muscle cells also affects the force of heart muscle contraction. When calcium levels are high, muscle cells contract with greater force, while when calcium levels are low, muscular contractions are less intense.

Last but not least, the heart muscle possesses an unusual quality termed automaticity, which allows it to produce electrical impulses independently of any external stimuli. If the SA node's electrical signals are interrupted, the heart can still beat because of this.

The heart couldn't function without the cardiac muscle, which allows for its contractions to be coordinated and rhythmic. Movement of ions, especially calcium ions, is crucial to the electrical and mechanical properties of heart muscle. Arrhythmias and heart failure are only two of the many heart disorders for which an understanding of cardiac muscle architecture and physiology is crucial.

Anatomy of the nervous system

The nervous system is an intricate web of cells and tissues that relays and processes information for the entire organism. The brain and spinal cord make up the central nervous system (CNS), while the nerves and ganglia outside of the CNS make up the peripheral nervous system (PNS). Learning about the structure of the nervous system is crucial for comprehending how the brain and nervous system work together.

The brain is the command center of the nervous system, and it regulates nearly every bodily function. The cerebral cortex, cerebellum, and brainstem are only a few of its many subdivisions. The cerebrum is the largest region of the brain and is in charge of thinking, moving voluntarily, and perceiving the world around you. The cerebellum, located near the brain's base, regulates equilibrium, coordination, and posture. Among the many automatic processes it regulates include respiration, heart rate, and blood pressure, the brainstem links the brain to the spinal cord.

The spinal cord is a collection of nerves that run the length of the spine from the brain stem to the tailbone. Its job is to relay messages from the brain to the rest of the body. The bones of the spinal column, called vertebrae, shield the spinal cord from harm.

The peripheral of the nervous system consists of two more divisions, namely the somatic and autonomic nervous systems. The somatic nervous system is responsible for the coordination of voluntary actions and the transmission of sensory information to the central nervous system. Breathing, heart rate, and digestion are instances of involuntary physiological activities regulated by the autonomic nervous system.

There are 31 spinal nerve pairs and 12 cranial nerve pairs that make up the PNS. These nerves relay messages from the central nervous system to the remainder of the body's sensory organs and motor systems. Information from sensory organs including the eyes, hearing, and skin is transmitted to the central nervous system via sensory nerves. Conversely, motor nerves provide messages from the central nervous system to the muscles and glands.

The brain and spinal cord are protected by three layers of tissue called the meninges, which are part of the nervous system. The brain and spinal cord are cushioned from shock and nourished by the cerebrospinal fluid, a clear, colorless liquid that circulates throughout the CNS.

distinct parts of the brain and spinal cord are responsible for distinct bodily processes; this complexity reflects the intricate nature of the nervous system's architecture. The peripheral nervous system relays sensory and motor impulses from the central nervous system to the remainder of the body. If you want to know how the nervous system works and how it communicates with everything else in the body, you need to know how it looks.

Physiology of the nervous system

The nervous system is a complex network of cells, tissues, and organs that coordinates and controls the body's responses to both internal and external stimuli. The nervous system consists of the central nervous system (CNS) and the peripheral nervous system (PNS). The nervous system consists of the brain and spinal cord as well as the nerves and ganglia outside of the CNS. Some of the many physical activities that the nervous system controls and regulates include movement, sensation, thought, and behavior.

Electrical and chemical impulses are transmitted throughout the nervous system to allow it to function. A neuron is a nerve cell that is specialized to produce and transmit electrical signals throughout the neurological system. Neurons are categorized according to their structure, function, and shape. Sensory neurons, motor neurons, and interneurons are the three main categories of neurons. Motor neurons transport messages from the central nervous system to the muscles and glands, while sensory neurons carry information from the sensory organs to the CNS. Interneurons are the cells in between sensory and motor neurons that process and integrate the information they receive.

Neurons and glial cells are the two primary cell types in the neurological system. While neurons are in charge of signal transmission and reception, glial cells are responsible for providing nourishment and defense for neurons. Astrocytes, oligodendrocytes, Schwann cells, and microglia are all examples of glial cells. Neurons rely on astrocytes for structural and metabolic support, myelin sheath is made by oligodendrocytes and Schwann cells, and microglia are engaged in the immunological response of the nervous system.

The nervous system is composed of the somatic nervous system and the autonomic nervous system, both of which control bodily functions. The autonomic nervous system manages automatic functions including heart rate, respiration, and digestion, while the somatic nervous system controls voluntary movements and sensory input. Both the sympathetic and parasympathetic nervous systems are subsets of the autonomic nervous system. The parasympathetic neural system regulates the body's "rest and digest" mechanism whereas the sympathetic nervous system controls the "fight or flight" reaction.

Neurotransmitters are chemicals released by nerve cells to facilitate communication between them. Neurons emit neurotransmitters, which are chemical messengers that bind to receptors on the receiving cell. Acetylcholine, dopamine, serotonin, and norepinephrine are all examples of neurotransmitters. Medications, hormones, and environmental conditions are only some of the ways in which neurotransmitter release can be altered.

The sleep-wake cycle is also controlled by the neurological system. Several brain areas, including the hypothalamus, thalamus, and brainstem, work together to control the body's sleep-wake cycle. The thalamus and brainstem are involved in controlling sleep stages, while the hypothalamus controls the circadian rhythm.

The nervous system is an elaborate and complicated network of tissues, cells, and organs that regulates the body's reactions to both internal and external stimuli. The central nervous system and the peripheral nervous system make up its entirety. The nervous system is the part of the body that sends and receives electrical and chemical signals to control things like movement, feeling, thought, and behavior. The sleep-wake cycle is regulated by the nervous system, which is made up of two functional divisions: the somatic nervous system and the autonomic nervous system.

Anatomy of the reproductive system

Reproduction relies on a vast system of interconnected organs, tissues, and hormones known as the reproductive system. Although the goal of both sexes is to have children, the way they go about doing so is different. The anatomy of the male and female reproductive systems is covered here.

Anatomy of the male reproductive system

The testicles, prostate gland, seminal vesicles, epididymis, vas deferens, and penis are all parts of the male reproductive system. The male reproductive system's main job is to make and move around sperm.

Testes

The scrotum houses two oval-shaped organs called the testes or testicles. Testes generate sperm and testosterone, the male sex hormone.

Epididymis

Along the back of each testicle is a long, coiled tube called the epididymis. Its job is to hold and nurture developing sperm.

Vas deferens

A muscular tube called the vas deferens connects the epididymis to the urethra. During ejaculation, it transports sperm from the epididymis to the urethra.

Prostate gland

The prostate gland is a walnut-sized organ found just in front of the rectum and below the bladder. Fluid created by this process is an integral component of semen.

Seminal vesicles

Two small glands found behind the bladder, called seminal vesicles, secrete a fluid that helps nourish and protect sperm.

Penis

The penis is an external organ that serves two purposes: urinating and sexual activity. The root, the shaft, and the glans are its three constituent parts.

Anatomy of the female reproductive system

The ovaries, uterus, fallopian tubes, cervix, and vagina are all parts of the female reproductive system. Feminine reproductive systems are primarily responsible for egg production, egg transportation, and fetal development.

Ovaries

Two almond-shaped glands sit on either side of the uterus; these are the ovaries. Eggs and female sex hormones are produced and released by them.

Fallopian tubes

The ovaries are connected to the uterus by two thin tubes called the fallopian tubes. The egg is moved from the ovary to the uterus by these structures.

Uterus

The uterus is a hollow, muscular structure found in the female pelvis. It ensures that a fertilized egg can successfully implant and grow into a baby.

Cervix

The cervix projects into the vagina as the lowest section of the uterus. It aids in preventing infection by directing menstrual blood away from the uterus and towards the vagina.

Vagina

The vagina is a muscular and elastic tube that leads from the cervix to the exterior of the body. It serves as both the birth canal and the place of sexual activity.

The human reproductive system is intricate and crucial to the continuation of the human race. Although the male and female reproductive systems seem different, they both serve the same basic purpose of creating and moving gametes. In order to properly diagnose and treat reproductive system problems, medical professionals must have a thorough understanding of the anatomy of the reproductive system.

Physiology of the reproductive system

The reproductive system's job is to ensure the survival of the species by creating new members of the species. The human reproductive system encompasses the anatomical structures responsible for reproduction in males and females. The male reproductive system comprises various anatomical structures, including the testes, epididymis, vas deferens, seminal vesicles, prostate gland, bulbourethral gland, urethra, and penis. The vagina, vulva, ovaries, uterus, fallopian tubes, cervix, and mammary glands make up the female reproductive system.

The female reproductive system creates eggs and offers a supportive environment for fetal development, while the male reproductive system produces and transports sperm cells. Hormones like testosterone, estrogen, and progesterone control reproduction.

The testes are the organs in males that generate sperm and the hormone testosterone. The epididymis is responsible for storing and maturing sperm after they have been created in the testes' seminiferous tubules. Ejaculation involves the release of sperm from the testes into the vas deferens, where they combine with fluids from the seminal vesicles, prostate gland, and bulbourethral gland to create semen.

The ovaries of a female reproductive system create and discharge eggs, which then make their way to the uterus via the fallopian tubes. A fetus develops from an implanted fertilized egg in the uterus. The cervix is the uterine orifice through which the vagina enters the body. During sexual activity, sperm cells are deposited close to the cervix when the penis enters the vagina. In the event of fertilization, a fertilized egg will implant in the uterine wall, where it will continue to develop into a fetus.

Hormones like estrogen and progesterone control the female reproductive system. In addition to its role in the menstrual cycle, estrogen is important for the growth of secondary sexual features like breasts and hips. Progesterone aids in uterine ripening and pregnancy maintenance after fertilization has taken place.

The uterine lining is shed and an egg is released from the ovary throughout the menstrual cycle, which is a series of changes in the female reproductive system. Estrogen, progesterone, follicle-stimulating hormone (FSH), and luteinizing hormone (LH) all have roles in regulating the cycle.

The follicles in the ovary, which contain the developing eggs, are stimulated to grow by FSH throughout the first part of the menstrual cycle. Follicles create more estrogen as they develop, causing the uterine lining to thicken in anticipation of an embryo being implanted there. Ovulation occurs when the levels of estrogen reach a critical point, at which point LH causes the ovary to release an egg.

If an egg is fertilized, it will implant in the uterus and start developing into a fetus. Menstruation occurs when the uterine lining is lost because estrogen and progesterone levels drop if fertilization does not take place.

Human reproduction relies on both the male and female reproductive systems, which are essential to the survival of the species. Healthcare providers cannot successfully diagnose and treat reproductive health disorders or provide age-appropriate care for patients without a firm grasp of the anatomy and physiology of these systems.

Anatomy of the respiratory system

The respiratory system allows air to enter the body and release carbon dioxide and oxygen. It is made up of various structures that cooperate to fulfill this crucial role. The nasal cavity, throat, voice box, windpipe, bronchi, and lungs all fall under this category.

The nasal cavity serves as the principal organ of the respiratory system, conditioning the air we breathe by preheating and humidifying it. Cilia and mucus in the nasal cavity filter the air and collect particles and germs that may otherwise enter the body. The pharynx, or throat, links the nasal and oral cavities with the esophagus and larynx.

The vocal cords are housed in the larynx, sometimes known as the "voice box," which is situated at the very top of the trachea. It's a safety device, too, sealing up the trachea to keep food and liquid from getting into the lungs as you swallow.

From the larynx to the bronchi lies a tube made of cartilage rings called the trachea or windpipe. The main airways that travel from the trachea to the lungs are called bronchi. The bronchioles are air passages within the lungs that are made of smooth muscle and cartilage and that branch off into even smaller air passages.

The lungs, the respiratory system's largest organ, perform the vital function of transferring oxygen and carbon dioxide from the air we breathe into the bloodstream. Alveoli are the microscopic air sacs that make up lungs; they are surrounded by capillaries. Capillaries take in oxygen from the air and distribute it throughout the body, whereas alveoli take in carbon dioxide from the blood and release it as exhaled breath.

Physiology of the respiratory system

Respiratory physiology is intricate, involving not only mechanical but also chemical processes. Inhaled air is filtered, warmed, and moistened as it travels through the nasal cavity after first entering the body through the mouth or nose. The vocal cords vibrate as air travels through the throat and larynx to create sound.

Air enters the lungs via the trachea and bronchi, and is then dispersed to the alveoli. Once oxygen from the air binds to hemoglobin molecules in red blood cells, it is carried throughout the body via a system of capillaries that surround the alveoli.

As a byproduct of cellular respiration, carbon dioxide enters the alveoli via diffusion from the blood and is expelled during expiration. The autonomic nervous system controls this process, which is affected by several variables, such as blood carbon dioxide and oxygen levels, blood pH, and lung volume.

The respiratory system does more than just exchange gases; it also helps control the acidity or alkalinity of the blood. Inadequate removal of carbon dioxide, an acid, can cause blood pH to drop. The amount of carbon dioxide expelled during breathing is a key factor in maintaining a healthy blood pH level.

The mucus lining the respiratory tract plays a role in the immune response by entrapping bacteria and debris. The mucus and debris that has become stuck in the respiratory system are cleared away by the cilia that line the airways, thereby reducing the risk of infection.

The respiratory system consists of the nasal cavity, the throat, the voice box, the windpipe, the trachea, the bronchi, and the lungs. The physiology of breathing includes the mechanical and chemical mechanisms that allow for the exchange of gases between the air and blood, the maintenance of a normal blood pH, and the activation of the immune system.

Anatomy of the skeletal system

Bones, cartilage, and ligaments make up the skeletal system, often called the musculoskeletal system. Its many roles include facilitating mobility, manufacturing blood cells, protecting essential organs, and giving structural support for the body. The skeletal system is described in great depth below.

Bones

The skeleton, of which the bones are the main component, serves as the body's supporting framework. Compact bone and spongy bone are the tissues that make them up. Bone can be either compact (which is solid) or spongy (which is porous and has small cavities filled with bone marrow). Bones might be long, short, flat, or uneven, and these characteristics are used to categorize them.

Joints

Where two or more bones meet is called a joint. Fibrous joints are the most common, followed by cartilaginous and then synovial joints. In contrast to mobile joints, fibrous joints are held together by stiff, inflexible fibrous tissue. Cartilage holds the bones of a joint together, allowing for a small range of motion. The majority of the body's joints are synovial joints, which are characterized by a joint capsule containing synovial fluid and allowing for frictionless movement.

Cartilage

Cartilage is a strong and pliable tissue that cushions the bones and facilitates easy movement at the joints. Cartilage is made up of cells called chondrocytes, which secrete a matrix that binds the cartilage together. The three primary forms of cartilage are hyaline cartilage, fibrocartilage, and elastic cartilage.

Ligaments

Strong bands of connective tissue called ligaments hold bones together and keep joints stable. Collagen fibers make up these structures, which can be found all over the body but especially in the joints (such as the knees, ankles, and wrists).

Tendons

Tough fibrous fibers called tendons join muscle to bone. Collagen fibers make up tendons, which play a crucial role in movement by transferring muscular tension to bone.

Bone marrow

The marrow in your bones is a fragile, sponge-like tissue. It generates RBCs, WBCs, and platelets (blood clotting cells).

Periosteum

A thin, fibrous membrane called the periosteum lines the exterior of bones. It's vital to bone growth and repair because it houses the blood arteries and nerves that bring nutrients to the bone.

The skeleton is an adaptive and ever-evolving mechanism that serves many functions. The study of its anatomy is fundamental to medical science, and the application of its physiology is critical to ensuring a person's continued good health.

Anatomy of the urinary system

The urinary system, also called the renal system, is in charge of flushing the body of waste and excess water. The urinary system includes the bladder, urethra, and ureters in addition to the two kidneys. Here we'll go through the anatomy of the urinary system and all its parts.

Kidneys

The kidneys, which are the size and form of beans, can be found on either side of the spine, below the rib cage. They are in charge of cleaning the blood of impurities and extra fluids. About a million of these microscopic filters, called nephrons, can be found in each kidney.

Ureters

Two thin tubes called ureters carry urine from the kidneys to the bladder. Through a process known as peristalsis, they move urine from the kidneys to the bladder.

Bladder

Urine is collected and stored in the bladder, a muscular sac with a hollow interior. It can be found in the pelvic region, below the belly button. As the bladder fills and empties, it is able to expand and shrink.

Urethra

The urethra is the tube that leads from the urinary bladder to the skin. The elimination of urine is a function of this organ. During ejaculation, the urethra also acts as a conduit for the male reproductive fluid known as semen.

There are a number of muscles, nerves, and blood vessels that contribute to the proper functioning of the urinary system. The detrusor muscle is a layer of muscle in the bladder wall responsible for ejecting pee. The urethra is surrounded by a ring of muscle called the external urethral sphincter, which plays a role in regulating urine flow. Having strong pelvic floor muscles is also crucial for continence.

The renal arteries are responsible for transporting blood to the kidneys, whilst the renal veins facilitate the return of blood to the heart. These blood vessels are among the several conduits that provide the urinary system with a blood supply. The autonomic nervous system governs the functioning of the urinary system, with its regulatory role in heart rate, digestive processes, and urine production.

The urinary system's major duty is waste removal and excess fluid elimination, but it also helps control blood pressure, maintain electrolyte balance, and produce hormones that increase red blood cell synthesis.

Waste and surplus fluids are flushed out of the body via the urinary system, a network of organs, muscles, nerves, and blood vessels. Medical personnel who treat patients with urinary tract diseases and disorders should have a firm grasp of urinary anatomy.

Physiology of the renal system

The kidneys, or urinary system, filter out metabolic wastes, excess water, and electrolytes to maintain a healthy balance in the body's fluids. The kidneys are the most obvious part of the renal system, but the ureters, bladder, and urethra are all part of it as well. Here, we'll go over the inner workings of the kidneys, such as their roles in filtration, reabsorption, secretion, and excretion.

Filtration

Filtration in the kidneys' nephrons is the first step in the renal system. About a million of these little filters, called nephrons, can be found in each kidney. The kidney is divided into tubules and glomeruli. The glomerulus is a system of capillaries that removes large and negatively charged particles from the blood. Capillaries act as filters, allowing only small molecules like water, glucose, and ions to enter the tubule. Proteins and red blood cells, both of which are much too massive to get through, therefore remain in the circulatory system.

Reabsorption

Reabsorption happens next in renal physiology, and it takes place in the tubules of the nephron. Reabsorption is the process by which beneficial elements that were filtered out of the blood are returned to it. The body relies on this process to keep its fluid and electrolyte levels stable. Glucose, amino acids, and a large portion of the filtered water are all substances that are reabsorbed.

Secretion

Secretion is the third stage of renal physiology. Hydrogen ions, creatinine, and medicines are only some of the molecules that are shuttled into the nephron tubules during the secretion process. The elimination of waste products and preservation of the body's acid-base balance are both aided by this process.

Excretion

The process of excretion is the last one in renal physiology. Urine is flushed out of the body by a process called excretion. The ureters connect the kidneys to the bladder and are responsible for the passage of urine. Urine is collected in the bladder and then sent out of the body via the urethra. Fluid consumption, electrolyte balance, and hormone modulation are just a few of the variables that affect the amount and chemical make-up of urine.

Controlling hormone levels

Hormones including ADH, aldosterone, and ANP (atrial natriuretic peptide) control the function of the kidneys. The pituitary gland secretes ADH in response to shifts in blood volume and osmolality. When the body is dehydrated, it aids in water conservation by acting on the kidneys to improve water reabsorption. Adrenal glands secrete aldosterone, which acts on the kidneys to boost sodium reabsorption and keep electrolyte levels stable. When blood volume increases, the atria of the heart secrete ANP. It reduces blood volume by stimulating the kidneys to release more salt and water.

The kidneys are responsible for regulating the fluid and electrolyte balance of the body. In the process of cleansing the blood, the kidneys recycle the good stuff and flush out the bad in the form of urine. Several hormones work together to keep the body's internal environment stable by controlling filtration, reabsorption, secretion, and excretion. In order to properly diagnose and treat renal diseases and abnormalities, medical personnel must have a firm grasp of renal physiology.

Anatomy of the eye

The human eye is an intricate organ that is vital to the process of seeing. It is surrounded by bone, muscle, and fat as it rests in the orbital cavity of the skull for protection. The anterior segment and the posterior segment are the two primary parts of the eye.

Cornea, iris, pupil, and lens together make up the anterior section of the eye, which is located in the front of the eye. The cornea is the transparent, dome-shaped front layer of the eye that aids in focusing light. Pupil size is regulated by the iris, the colorful portion of the eye that sits in the optical pathway of the eyeball. Light is focused onto the retina via the lens, a transparent structure located behind the iris.

The posterior segment of the eye, situated at the posterior region, consists of the retina, optic nerve, and vitreous humor. The retina, a thin layer of tissue located at the posterior part of the eye, has a vast number of photoreceptor cells. These cells play a crucial role in the process of converting incoming light into electrical signals, which are then transmitted to the brain. The optic nerve serves as the conduit via which the retina establishes a connection with the brain, facilitated by a complex network of nerve fibers. The region situated between the lens and the retina is occupied by a translucent gel-like substance known as the vitreous humor.

Eyelids, eyelashes, and tear ducts are only few of the supplementary structures that surround the eye. The eyelashes and eyelids work together to prevent dust and other debris from entering the eye. The tears produced by the tear ducts assist keep the eye's surface lubricated and clean.

The ophthalmic artery, which originates from the internal carotid artery, and the central retinal artery are just two of the many arteries that bring oxygenated blood to the eye.

Each component of the eye's intricate and highly specialized anatomy serves a crucial purpose in the health of the visual system as a whole. In order to properly diagnose and treat a wide variety of ocular diseases and disorders, knowledge of eye anatomy is crucial.

Eye physiology

Physiologically speaking, seeing clearly requires a number of different structures and mechanisms to work in concert with one another. Upon entering the ocular organ, light undergoes a process of convergence onto the retinal surface, where it undergoes a transformation into electrical signals. These electrical impulses are subsequently transmitted to the brain through the optic nerve. The process involves the participation of various ocular structures, namely the cornea, lens, iris, ciliary body, retina, and optic nerve.

The cornea is the eye's protective outer covering, and it also plays a role in focusing incoming light. The lens, which sits just below the iris, is a transparent, malleable structure that may alter its form to better concentrate light onto the retina. The iris, the eye's colorful portion, regulates how much light enters the eye by changing the diameter of the pupil. In order to concentrate on things at varying distances, the ciliary body, which is located beneath the eye, changes the lens's shape.

Both rods and cones, found in the retina at the rear of the eye, are essential for vision. Vision in dim light is handled by rods, which are sensitive to light intensity, while color perception is handled by cones, which are sensitive to light wavelength. The rods and cones receive incoming light, process it into electrical signals, and send them via the optic nerve to the brain.

The visual images you see in your mind's eye are actually electrical impulses sent from your retina to your brain. The brain converts these impulses into images, allowing us to take in our visual environment.

The eye's physiology also includes accommodation, the process of changing the focal length of the lens in order to concentrate on things at varying distances. The ciliary muscles contract and relax to alter the lens's shape and thus the eye's ability to focus on things at varying distances.

Convergence, the ability of the eyes to move together to focus on a single object, is another physiological feature of the eye. The eye muscles known as the extraocular muscles must work together to do this.

Adaptation, the eyes' ability to adjust to variations in light intensity, is also a part of the eye's physiology. Pupil dilation and retinal rod and cone sensitivity regulation are involved in this process.

Physiologically speaking, seeing clearly requires a number of different structures and mechanisms to work in concert with one another. The ability to diagnose and cure visual issues as well as maintain healthy eyes requires knowledge of eye physiology.

Anatomy of the ear

The ear, which aids in hearing and balance, is a delicate and intricate organ. It has an external ear, a middle ear, and an internal ear. Each component contributes significantly to the overall function of hearing and cooperates with the others to provide auditory signals to the brain.

The part of the ear that sticks out from the side of the head is called the outer ear, auricle, or pinna. Its cartilage structure, which is covered by skin, collects and directs sound waves into the ear canal. The ear canal, or external auditory meatus, is a tiny passageway linking the external ear to the middle ear. To keep the middle ear safe from bacteria and dust, the canal is coated with hair and wax-secreting glands.

Behind the eardrum is a tiny space called the middle ear, which is filled with air. The ossicles are three little bones responsible for conducting sound vibrations from the eardrum to the cochlea. The ossicles are made up of three smaller bones: the malleus, incus, and stapes. The Eustachian tube is a small tube that runs from the middle ear to the base of the neck. The Eustachian tube drains fluid and avoids infection by keeping the middle ear at a constant pressure with the surroundings.

The labyrinth is the collective name for the intricate network of canals and chambers that make up the inner ear, which is situated at the base of the brain. The cochlea and the vestibular system are its two primary components. The cochlea serves as the auditory organ, wherein sound waves are converted into electrical impulses by the minuscule hair cells. These electrical signals are subsequently transmitted to the brain through the auditory nerve. The vestibular system, which detects head movement and position, consists of three semicircular canals and two otolith organs.

The snail-shaped cochlea contains three primary chambers, each with its own specialized hair cells. The basilar membrane, which extends the length of the cochlea, is lined with rows of hair cells. When sound waves reach the cochlea, they force the hair cells there to vibrate, which in turn activates the auditory nerve fibers. The brainstem receives electrical impulses via the auditory nerve and interprets them as sound.

The utricle and saccule are the two otolith organs that make up the vestibular system, together with the three semicircular canals. The otolith organs are responsible for the detection of linear acceleration and gravity, whereas the semicircular canals are responsible for detecting rotational motion of the head. The cupula, also known as the otolithic membrane, is a gel-like substance in which hair cells are embedded in each of these organs. Gel and hair cells are displaced as the head moves, sending signals to the brainstem that aid in equilibrium and navigation.

The outer ear, the middle ear, and the inner ear make up the ear, a complicated organ. The middle ear, which houses the ossicles and aids in sound wave transmission to the inner ear, receives sound waves from the outer ear and directs them into the ear canal. The vestibular system, which is in charge of maintaining balance and spatial orientation, and the cochlea, which is responsible for hearing, are both found in the inner ear. The body's ability to perceive and react to auditory and vestibular cues depends on the coordinated efforts of these components.

Physiology of the ear

The ear is a highly sophisticated sensory organ that is essential for hearing and equilibrium. The ear has an external ear, a middle ear, and an internal ear. The many components of the ear work together to help with hearing and equilibrium in their own special ways.

In order to hear and keep our balance, our ears undergo a series of intricate physiological processes. The pinna is responsible for directing sound waves into the external auditory canal. The ossicles in the middle ear move in response to the vibration of the eardrum, which is caused by the sound waves. In this way, the sound waves are amplified before being sent to the cochlea in the inner ear. The cochlea contains minuscule hair cells that convert vibrations into electrical signals, which are then transmitted through the auditory nerve to the brain. These electrical impulses are translated by the brain into audible sound.

The ear is important for more than just hearing sounds; it also helps with balance. Changes in head position and movement are sensed by the vestibular system in the inner ear. The fluid in the semicircular canals and the otolith organs moves when we do, stimulating the hair cells there. Signals from this stimulation reach the brain, assisting with both equilibrium and direction.

The ear is a sophisticated sensory organ that is essential for hearing and equilibrium. The outer ear acts as a receiver for incoming sound waves and a barrier against dust and bacteria. The sound waves are amplified in the middle ear before being sent to the inner ear. The inner ear processes sound waves into electrical signals that are transmitted to the brain, and it also houses the sensory receptors responsible for hearing and balance.

The Nose's Anatomy

The nose is a vital part of the respiratory system, allowing air to enter the lungs and providing us with our sense of smell. There are both visible and invisible components to the nose's anatomy. Everything that can be seen when you look at a person's nose is considered part of the external nose. The nasal cavity, which is split in two by the nasal septum, and the sinuses make up the nose's interior structures.

Mucous membranes and tiny hair-like projections called cilia line the inside of the nasal cavity, which is filled with air. Respiratory epithelium is a particular form of tissue that lines the nasal cavity and contributes to the humidification and warming of inhaled air. Olfactory receptors are specialized cells found in the respiratory epithelium that are responsible for perceiving odors.

The nasal septum is a thin partition made of cartilage and bone that divides the nasal cavity into the left and right sides. It is well supplied with blood and lined with respiratory epithelium. The sinuses are four air-filled cavities in the skull bones close to the nasal cavity. Mucous membranes coat them, and they connect to the nasal cavity through tiny orifices.

Bone, cartilage, and skin compose the exterior structures of the nose. The nasal bones create the nose's bridge, while cartilage makes up the nose's lower third. The thin skin that lines the nose is moisturized and kept moist by the glands of the same name.

Several auxiliary structures aid in the operation of the nose. The nasal turbinates, which are bony protrusions lined with mucous membranes, play a role in the filtration and warming of air in the nasal passages. Nasal conchae, which are folds of tissue, have a similar function by filtering and moistening the air.

The nose isn't just important for breathing; it's also where we take in our surroundings through our sense of smell. Odors are picked up by the olfactory receptors in the nasal cavity and sent on to the brain via the olfactory nerve. The olfactory nerve is a collection of specialized nerve cells in the nasal roof that can identify a wide variety of odors.

The nose is a highly specialized organ with an intricate architecture that includes both exterior and interior elements. Because of its importance to breathing and smelling, the nose is an integral element of the human body.

Anatomy of the nose

The nose is a vital part of the respiratory system, allowing air to enter the lungs and providing us with our sense of smell. There are both visible and invisible components to the nose's anatomy. Everything that can be seen when you look at a person's nose is considered part of the external nose. The nasal cavity, which is split in two by the nasal septum, and the sinuses make up the nose's interior structures.

Mucous membranes and tiny hair-like projections called cilia line the inside of the nasal cavity, which is filled with air. Respiratory epithelium is a particular form of tissue that lines the nasal cavity and contributes to the humidification and warming of inhaled air. Olfactory receptors are specialized cells found in the respiratory epithelium that are responsible for perceiving odors.

The nasal septum is a thin partition made of cartilage and bone that divides the nasal cavity into the left and right sides. It is well supplied with blood and lined with respiratory epithelium. The sinuses are four air-filled cavities in the skull bones close to the nasal cavity. Mucous membranes coat them, and they connect to the nasal cavity through tiny orifices.

Bone, cartilage, and skin compose the exterior structures of the nose. The nasal bones create the nose's bridge, while cartilage makes up the nose's lower third. The thin skin that lines the nose is moisturized and kept moist by the glands of the same name.

Several auxiliary structures aid in the operation of the nose. The nasal turbinates, which are bony protrusions lined with mucous membranes, play a role in the filtration and warming of air in the nasal passages. Nasal conchae, which are folds of tissue, have a similar function by filtering and moistening the air.

The nose isn't just important for breathing; it's also where we take in our surroundings through our sense of smell. Odors are picked up by the olfactory receptors in the nasal cavity and sent on to the brain via the olfactory nerve. The olfactory nerve is a collection of specialized nerve cells in the nasal roof that can identify a wide variety of odors.

The nose is a highly specialized organ with an intricate architecture that includes both exterior and interior elements. Because of its importance to breathing and smelling, the nose is an integral element of the human body.

Physiology of the nose

Our ability to breathe and smell depends on the nose, which serves an important function in the respiratory system. Its physiology consists of a network of interconnected structures and processes.

Before it reaches the lungs, the air we breathe must first pass through the nasal passages, where it is cleaned, warmed, and humidified. The mucous membranes lining the nasal canal create mucus, which acts as a filter by capturing dust and other airborne particles. Once the mucus reaches the back of the throat, it is either ingested or ejected by coughing or sneezing by microscopic hair-like structures called cilia.

The nose is important for more than just filtering the air we breathe; it's also where our sense of smell is processed. The olfactory system, which can detect and interpret smells, is found in the nasal cavity's upper esophagus. When we take a deep breath in, molecules from the air trigger olfactory epithelial cells, which in turn send signals to the brain, which we interpret as odors.

The nasal cavity communicates with the sinuses, which are air-filled cavities in the skull bones close to the nose. The mucus produced by the sinuses helps to warm and humidify the air and reduces pressure inside of the skull. Sinus discomfort, pressure, and other symptoms can develop, however, when the sinuses become clogged or infected.

The nose also controls the amount of air that enters the lungs, which is an essential function. The nasal passages are equipped with specific cells that can detect variations in temperature and humidity, allowing them to expand or contract to regulate the volume of air entering the lungs.

In addition to its physiological roles, the nose is also vulnerable to a host of disorders and diseases. Breathing problems and other symptoms might result from the nose's inability to operate normally due to congestion, inflammation, or infections like sinusitis. Nasal symptoms including a runny nose, sneezing, and itching can also be caused by allergies and other immune system problems.

There is a lot going on in the background of the nose's physiology that allows us to breathe and smell. Better care for nose and respiratory disorders can be provided by medical practitioners who have a firm grasp on these functions and how they may be impacted by disease and other circumstances.

Anatomy of the tongue

The tongue is the most important organ in the human body for both tasting and speaking. It's a complicated structure made up of several tissues and muscles that all serve certain purposes.

There are two distinct sections of the tongue: the front, called the oral tongue, and the back, called the pharyngeal tongue. The papillae on the oral tongue are the taste buds that you can feel when you put your tongue out in your mouth. The pharyngeal tongue assists in swallowing and is placed at the very back of the throat.

The pink mucous membrane covering the tongue is made up of many layers of cells. Located on the epithelium, the top layer of cells, are the taste receptors. The ability to distinguish between sweet, sour, salty, and bitter is the job of taste buds.

Connective tissue containing blood arteries and nerves lies beneath the epithelium. Underneath this sheet of connective tissue lie the tongue's muscles. The tongue is moved by eight muscles, four intrinsic and four extrinsic.

Tongue size and form are controlled by four intrinsic muscles found deep within the tongue. The names of these muscles are the transversus linguae, the verticalis linguae, the transversus oblique, and the longitudinalis superior and inferior.

The four muscles on the outside of the tongue are what actually do the work of moving the tongue in and out of the mouth. The genioglossus, hyoglossus, styloglossus, and palatoglossus are the names given to these groups of muscles.

The role of the tongue in communication cannot be understated. Tongue movement contributes to the production of speech sounds. Sounds can be made by placing the tongue in a variety of locations in the mouth.

The tongue is also crucial to the success of the swallowing process. The ball of food and saliva that results from chewing is termed a bolus. The tongue then moves the bolus to the rear of the mouth, where it is pushed into the pharynx and swallowed.

The tongue has many crucial purposes beyond taste, speaking, and swallowing. The continual motion and removal of food particles helps maintain a clean mouth and teeth. Its ability to dissipate heat through the tongue's surface also contributes to maintaining a healthy internal body temperature.

Multiple types of tissue and muscles make up the tongue, making it an intricate organ. It controls your sense of taste, as well as your ability to speak and swallow. The tongue is an integral organ, and it is critical for overall health that it work normally.

Physiology of the tongue

The tongue, a muscular organ in the mouth, is an important part of the body for both digestion and sensation. The tongue is covered in a mucous membrane that contains taste buds, which are important for detecting distinct flavors, and is made up of skeletal muscle tissue that allows it to move in different directions.

The tongue's primary role is to facilitate the mechanical breakdown of meals. During mastication, the process of reducing food to smaller pieces by chewing and grinding it with the teeth, the tongue plays an important role in manipulating and mixing the food. The bolus, a small, easily ingested mass of food, is formed in part by the tongue.

The tongue is involved in the sensation of taste in addition to its digestive functions. Thousands of taste buds, specialized sensory organs, are located on the tongue's surface and are responsible for perceiving various flavors. Sweet, sour, bitter, salty, and umami are the five basic flavors that make up the human tastebuds. Taste buds are made up of groups of cells that each have their own receptors for a certain flavor. Flavor is perceived when certain taste receptors on the tongue are activated by molecules in food or drink and transmit messages to the brain.

The tongue also has a hand in the articulation of words. The tongue, along with the lips and teeth, helps to create the wide range of sounds that make up human speech. Consonant sounds, which involve precise movements of the tongue and other structures in the mouth, put the tongue in the spotlight.

The tongue also plays a crucial role in promoting good oral hygiene. Tooth decay and gum disease are just two of the dental issues that can be avoided with a little help from the tongue's cleaning abilities. The tongue's surface is covered with tiny projections called papillae that aid in creating friction when the tongue comes into contact with food or other oral surfaces. The rubbing action eliminates trash and germs from the tongue and its surrounding areas.

One more thing: the tongue can help you feel things. The tongue is a very sensitive organ, capable of perceiving both temperature and texture differences. Because of this heightened awareness, we are able to avoid harm by taking precautions around hot food or sharp items.

The tongue is a multifaceted organ that serves numerous critical roles in the body. Its many uses range from assisting digestion to detecting odors to making speaking sounds to ensuring good dental hygiene to sensing changes in temperature and texture. If you want to keep your mouth and body in tip-top shape, it helps to have a firm grasp on the tongue's anatomy and physiology.

Medications

Antihypertensive drugs

Hypertension, or high blood pressure, can be treated with antihypertensive medications. Worldwide, a sizable percentage of the population deals with high blood pressure. High blood pressure occurs when the blood pressure against the artery walls is too great. Many major health issues, including cardiovascular disease, stroke, and kidney failure, can result from this. Blood pressure can be lowered and the likelihood of these side effects mitigated by antihypertensive medication.

Different kinds of antihypertensive medications accomplish their desired effects in various ways. Diuretics, beta-blockers, angiotensin-converting enzyme (ACE) inhibitors, angiotensin receptor blockers (ARBs), calcium channel blockers, and renin inhibitors are the most widely prescribed groups of antihypertensive medications.

In the early stages of treating hypertension, diuretics are frequently used. By stimulating urination, they help the body get rid of extra sodium and water. As a result, there is less fluid pushing against the walls of the blood arteries, and the pressure there is reduced. Hydrochlorothiazide, furosemide, and spironolactone are just a few examples of diuretics.

Adrenaline causes the heart to beat quicker and harder; beta blockers counteract this effect. Beta blockers lower blood pressure by decreasing the heart's pace and the force with which it contracts. Metoprolol, atenolol, and propranolol are all examples of beta blockers.

Angiotensin-converting enzyme (ACE) inhibitors lower blood pressure by preventing the generation of the hormone angiotensin II. Blood pressure can rise because angiotensin II causes blood vessels to constrict. ACE inhibitors work to dilate blood arteries and reduce blood pressure by inhibiting the formation of angiotensin-converting enzyme (ACE). Lisinopril, enalapril, and ramipril are all types of ACE inhibitors.

In contrast to ACE inhibitors, which work by preventing the formation of angiotensin II, ARBs prevent the activity of angiotensin II. As a result, blood vessels relax and blood pressure drops. Losartan, valsartan, and candesartan are all examples of ARBs.

The cochlea contains minuscule hair cells that convert vibrations into electrical signals, which are then transmitted through the auditory nerve to the brain. As a result, blood vessel relaxation and weaker heart contractions lower blood pressure. Amlodipine, nifedipine, and verapamil are all examples of calcium channel blockers.

Renin inhibitors are a relatively new type of antihypertensive medication that inhibits renin, an enzyme necessary for the synthesis of angiotensin II. Renin inhibitors work to dilate blood vessels and reduce blood pressure by decreasing the body's synthesis of this hormone. Aliskiren is the only renin inhibitor currently in use.

Although antihypertensive medication is often successful in reducing blood pressure, it is not without risk of side effects. Dizziness, lethargy, headaches, and nausea are all common negative reactions to antihypertensive medication. Some antihypertensive medications, including beta blockers, have the potential to lower blood pressure, increasing the risk of fainting or dizziness.

Patients should strictly adhere to their healthcare provider's instructions when it comes to taking antihypertensive medications. Stopping antihypertensive medicines suddenly might cause a severe spike in blood pressure, so patients shouldn't do so without first talking to their doctor.

High blood pressure is typically treated with antihypertensive medication. Different kinds of antihypertensive medications work in different ways and have different potential negative effects. Although these treatments tend to be well-tolerated, they require close monitoring and management due to the possibility of serious side effects and drug interactions.

Antiplatelets

Antiplatelet drugs are a class of medicines that stop platelets from clumping together, a vital step in the blood clotting process. Blood clots can be avoided and the risk of cardiovascular events like heart attacks and strokes reduced with antiplatelet medication. These medications are effective because they either prevent platelets from becoming activated (like thromboxane and ADP) or they impede the action of platelet-aggregating substances.

Commonly used in low doses (81 mg/day), aspirin is the most widely prescribed antiplatelet medication. Aspirin prevents platelets from sticking together by blocking the synthesis of thromboxane A2, a powerful platelet-aggregating agent. Aspirin prevents platelet aggregation and the formation of blood clots by inhibiting the synthesis of thromboxane A2. Antiplatelet medications also include clopidogrel, prasugrel, ticagrelor, and dipyridamole.

Thienopyridine medicines like clopidogrel, prasugrel, and ticagrelor function by irreversibly inhibiting the P2Y12 receptor on platelets, therefore limiting ADP-mediated platelet activation. Patients with acute coronary syndromes, such as unstable angina and myocardial infarction, and patients with stents to prevent stent thrombosis often take these medications in conjunction with aspirin for the prevention of cardiovascular events.

Dipyridamole is a phosphodiesterase inhibitor that decreases platelet aggregation by raising cyclic adenosine monophosphate (cAMP) levels. Patients who have already suffered a stroke or TIA often take aspirin in addition to dipyridamole for secondary stroke prevention.

Although antiplatelet medication has a high rate of patient acceptance and is seldom associated with serious adverse events, it does raise the risk of bleeding, which is especially concerning for patients undergoing invasive operations or who have a history of bleeding disorders. Antiplatelet therapy's most common adverse effect is bleeding, which can vary from moderate bruising to life-threatening hemorrhage. Patients on antiplatelet medications should be watched for bruises, nosebleeds, and blood in the toilet. Depending on the severity of bleeding, antiplatelet medication may need to be stopped temporarily or permanently.

Blood clots and cardiovascular events can be avoided, in large part, thanks to antiplatelet medicines. Most people think of aspirin when they hear "antiplatelet drug," but there are actually several more that work just as well. Although antiplatelet medication has a high rate of patient acceptance and is seldom associated with serious adverse events, it does raise the risk of bleeding, which is especially concerning for patients undergoing invasive operations or who have a history of bleeding disorders. If a patient is on an antiplatelet medication and experiences bleeding, the medication may need to be stopped, either temporarily or permanently.

Thrombolvtics

Drugs belonging to the thrombolytic or fibrinolytic class are used to break up clots in the blood. Clots in the blood vessels can cause major health problems, including heart attack, stroke, and pulmonary embolism, if the blood flow is blocked. Thrombolytics help break down clots and get blood flowing again by stimulating the body's own natural clot-dissolving system.

Mechanism of Action

Thrombolytics function by transforming the inactive precursor plasminogen into the active enzyme plasmin, which cleaves the fibrin that supports blood clots. The liver generates plasminogen, which then travels through the body's bloodstream. Plasminogen is integrated into a clot during its formation and is converted to plasmin if thrombolytic medicines are administered. The fibrin strands in the clot are subsequently broken down by plasmin, resulting in the clot's disintegration.

Indications

Thrombolytics are used to treat several illnesses brought on by blood clots. These include acute myocardial infarction (heart attack), deep vein thrombosis (DVT), pulmonary embolism (PE), and acute ischemic stroke. Since rapid restoration of blood flow is crucial in emergency conditions where organ damage or death could result from a lack of blood flow, thrombolytics are most effective when administered immediately after the beginning of symptoms.

Types of Thrombolytics

Thrombolytic medicines such as streptokinase, urokinase, alteplase, reteplase, and tenecteplase are currently available. The bacterial streptokinase and urokinase are the only naturally occurring plasminogen activators; the rest are modified forms of human tPA. Alteplase has been demonstrated to be successful in treating acute ischemic stroke, acute myocardial infarction, and pulmonary embolism, making it the most widely used thrombolytic medication.

Administration

Intravenous administration of thrombolytics can be done either a peripheral vein or a central line. The drug's dosage is determined by the patient's weight and the seriousness of their disease. After an initial bolus injection, thrombolytics are often administered as a continuous infusion over the course of several hours. Because bleeding is a common adverse effect of thrombolytics, patients are closely watched during treatment.

Contraindications and Precautions

There are a number of factors that must be taken into account before deciding to give a patient a thrombolytic medication. Patients who are not good candidates for thrombolytic therapy include those who have undergone recent surgery or trauma, have a history of bleeding disorders, are pregnant, or have uncontrolled hypertension. Patients having a history of peptic ulcer disease, cerebral hemorrhage, or recent trauma are at an increased risk for bleeding and should be treated with caution when receiving thrombolytics.

Side Effects

Bleeding is the most common adverse effect of thrombolytic therapy and can happen anywhere in the body. Patients who are older, have a history of bleeding problems, or have other medical factors that enhance the risk of bleeding are at a higher risk of experiencing bleeding within the first few hours after therapy. Allergic reactions, fever, nausea, vomiting, and hypotension are among possible reactions to thrombolytic therapy.

Anticoagulants

Blood thinners, or anticoagulants, are drugs that reduce the likelihood of blood clots forming or expanding in the circulatory system. Patients with a history of clot-forming conditions, such as atrial fibrillation, deep vein thrombosis (DVT), pulmonary embolism, or those who have recently suffered a cardiovascular event, are popular candidates for these medications. Anticoagulants assist keep the blood from clotting dangerously by interfering with the body's normal coagulation mechanism.

Anticoagulants come in a variety of forms, each with its own mode of action and set of advantages. Oral anticoagulants and injectable anticoagulants are the two primary types of anticoagulants.

Anticoagulants can be taken orally, and some examples are warfarin, dabigatran, apixaban, and rivaroxaban. The most widely prescribed oral anticoagulant is warfarin, also known as Coumadin. Blood coagulation is slowed because production of vitamin K is reduced. Newer oral anticoagulants include dabigatran, apixaban, and rivaroxaban directly suppress certain blood clotting factors. Compared to warfarin, these drugs have fewer food restrictions and require less regular monitoring.

Among the injectable anticoagulants are heparin and LMWHs like enoxaparin and dalteparin. When a patient has a life-threatening medical condition such a pulmonary embolism or deep vein thrombosis, these drugs are commonly utilized in an emergency setting at a hospital. They prevent blood clots from forming and are administered subcutaneously.

Blood clots are potentially fatal, but anticoagulants can save lives if taken in time. Bleeding, ranging from minor bruising to serious hemorrhaging, is the most often reported adverse effect of anticoagulants. Patients on anticoagulants should be regularly monitored for signs of bleeding, and those who encounter any unusual bleeding or bruises should be urged to seek emergency medical attention. To counteract the anticoagulant and assist halt bleeding, reversal medicines such vitamin K or protamine sulfate may be given.

Anticoagulants raise the danger of drug interactions in addition to the risk of bleeding. To avoid potentially dangerous drug interactions, patients taking anticoagulants should tell their healthcare provider about all drugs, supplements, and herbal remedies they are currently taking.

People who are at risk of developing life-threatening blood clots must take anticoagulants. While there are hazards associated with these drugs, they can be mitigated with careful monitoring and patient education.

Antiarrhythmies

Antiarrhythmics are drugs used to treat abnormal heart rhythms, also known as arrhythmias. These drugs work by altering the electrical properties of the heart to regulate its rhythm. Arrhythmias can be caused by various factors, including drug toxicity, heart disease, electrolyte imbalances, and genetic factors. Antiarrhythmic drugs are classified into four classes based on their mechanism of action.

Class I antiarrhythmics are sodium channel blockers that work by slowing the conduction of electrical impulses through the heart. There are three subclasses of Class I antiarrhythmics:

1A drugs (e.g., quinidine, procainamide) prolong the duration of the action potential and decrease the rate of depolarization. These drugs are used to treat atrial fibrillation, ventricular tachycardia, and other types of arrhythmias.

1B drugs (e.g., lidocaine, mexiletine) shorten the duration of the action potential and increase the rate of depolarization. These drugs are used to treat ventricular arrhythmias, especially those associated with acute myocardial infarction.

1C drugs (e.g., flecainide, propafenone) have little effect on the duration of the action potential but markedly decrease the rate of depolarization. These drugs are used to treat supraventricular tachycardia and ventricular arrhythmias.

Class II antiarrhythmics are beta-blockers that work by blocking the effects of adrenaline on the heart. These drugs slow the heart rate, decrease the force of contraction, and reduce the workload of the heart. Class II antiarrhythmics are used to treat atrial fibrillation, ventricular tachycardia, and other types of arrhythmias.

Class III antiarrhythmics are potassium channel blockers that prolong the duration of the action potential and delay repolarization. These drugs increase the refractory period and decrease the excitability of the heart, which helps to prevent arrhythmias. There are several drugs in this class, including amiodarone, dronedarone, sotalol, and dofetilide. These drugs are used to treat various types of arrhythmias, including atrial fibrillation, ventricular tachycardia, and atrial flutter.

Class IV antiarrhythmics are calcium channel blockers that work by blocking the flow of calcium into the heart cells. This decreases the force of contraction and slows the heart rate, which helps to treat arrhythmias. There are two drugs in this class: verapamil and diltiazem. These drugs are used to treat supraventricular tachycardia and atrial fibrillation.

In addition to the four classes of antiarrhythmics, there are other drugs that are used to treat arrhythmias. These include adenosine, which is used to treat paroxysmal supraventricular tachycardia, and digoxin, which is used to control the heart rate in patients with atrial fibrillation.

Antiarrhythmic drugs can have serious side effects, including proarrhythmic effects that can actually worsen arrhythmias. They can also cause hypotension, bradycardia, and other cardiovascular effects. Therefore, they should only be used under the supervision of a physician with experience in the management of arrhythmias.

Diuretics

Diuretics are a group of medications that are used to increase urine output by the kidneys, leading to a reduction in fluid volume in the body. They are commonly prescribed for conditions such as hypertension, heart failure, liver disease, and kidney disease. Diuretics work by inhibiting the reabsorption of sodium and water in the kidneys, leading to an increase in urine output and a decrease in blood volume.

There are three main classes of diuretics: thiazide diuretics, loop diuretics, and potassium-sparing diuretics. Thiazide diuretics, such as hydrochlorothiazide, are often used as first-line therapy for hypertension and can also be used for edema associated with heart failure. Loop diuretics, such as furosemide, are used for more severe edema and in acute settings such as pulmonary edema. Potassium-sparing diuretics, such as spironolactone, are used in combination with other diuretics to prevent potassium depletion.

Thiazide diuretics work by inhibiting sodium reabsorption in the distal convoluted tubule of the kidney, leading to an increase in urine output. They are effective at reducing blood pressure and can also be used to treat edema. However, they can cause hypokalemia, hyponatremia, and hypercalcemia as side effects.

Loop diuretics work by inhibiting sodium and chloride reabsorption in the ascending loop of Henle in the kidney. They are effective at reducing fluid overload and pulmonary edema, but can also cause hypokalemia, hyponatremia, and hypocalcemia as side effects. Loop diuretics are often used in acute settings such as heart failure exacerbations or pulmonary edema.

Potassium-sparing diuretics work by blocking the action of aldosterone in the collecting duct of the kidney, leading to increased sodium and water excretion while sparing potassium. They are often used in combination with other diuretics to prevent potassium depletion, but can also cause hyperkalemia as a side effect.

Diuretics are generally well-tolerated, but they can cause electrolyte imbalances and dehydration if not monitored closely. Patients taking diuretics should have regular monitoring of their electrolyte levels and kidney function. It is also important to monitor blood pressure and symptoms of fluid overload or dehydration.

Diuretics are an important class of medications used to treat conditions such as hypertension, heart failure, and kidney disease. There are three main classes of diuretics, each with its own mechanism of action and side effect profile. Close monitoring of electrolytes and kidney function is necessary when taking diuretics to prevent complications.

Analgesics

Analgesics are drugs that reduce pain by altering how a person experiences the stimuli that are causing it. They have the ability to relieve both acute pain—such as that caused by an injury or surgery—and chronic pain—such as that caused by cancer or arthritis. There are two types of analgesics: those that are opioids and those that are not.

Non-opioid Analgesics

Non-opioid analgesics are painkillers that have no effect whatsoever on the central nervous system. These over-the-counter (OTC) drugs are widely accessible and typically the first that people turn to when they need relief from mild to moderate pain. Some analgesics that don't contain opioids include the following:

Acetaminophen

It has been demonstrated that the widely used non-opioid analgesic paracetamol is effective in relieving mild to severe pain. Numerous unpleasant illnesses, such as toothaches, headaches, and menstrual cramps, are routinely treated with it. Acetaminophen can be acquired without a prescription and is regarded to be safe for the majority of individuals when used at the prescribed levels.

Nonsteroidal anti-inflammatory drugs (NSAIDs)

Non-steroidal anti-inflammatory medicines, or NSAIDs, are analgesics that do not include opioids but are nonetheless effective in reducing inflammation and alleviating pain. They are widely used to relieve menstrual cramps, arthritic pain, and other types of discomfort. Non-steroidal anti-inflammatory drugs (NSAIDs) include medications including ibuprofen, naproxen, and aspirin. Nonsteroidal anti-inflammatory medicines (NSAIDs) can be acquired over-the-counter or without a prescription, depending on the dosage and intensity.

Opioid Analgesics

Opioid analgesics are drugs that work with specific central nervous system receptors to lessen or completely eliminate the perception of pain. Patients with moderate to severe pain, such as those affected by cancer or surgical operations, are administered these. Opioids are only available with a doctor's prescription and are subject to strict controls because of the significant risk of abuse and addiction. Here are a few instances of opioid analgesics:

Morphine

A strong opioid analgesic, morphine is frequently used in medical settings to alleviate severe pain. It is frequently given orally or intravenously, and its effects may last for several hours. In addition to causing side effects such sleepiness, nausea, and constipation, morphine has a high potential for abuse and addiction.

Oxycodone

Strong opioid analgesic oxycodone is often prescribed to treat moderate to severe pain. Its efficacy varies between 50 and 100 percent. It comes in immediate-release and extended-release forms and is usually taken alongside paracetamol, which offers further pain relief. Oxycodone is only legally available with a doctor's prescription due to its high risk of abuse and addiction.

Fentanyl

A strong opioid analgesic known as fentanyl is used to treat extreme pain, such as the kind brought on by cancer treatment or surgical procedures. It is available for purchase and comes in a range of formulations, including patches, injections, and lozenges. Fentanyl is only legally available with a doctor's prescription due to its high risk of abuse and addiction.

An important class of drugs that are used to manage pain is called analgesics. Non-opioid analgesics are often used to treat mild to moderate pain, whereas opioid analgesics are typically designated for the treatment of moderate to severe pain. Despite the fact that these drugs are highly effective, they must be used with considerable caution due to the risk of abuse and addiction. It is crucial to take the drug exactly as prescribed, both in terms of dosage and frequency, and to seek expert assistance if any unintended side effects manifest.

Anticonvulsants

A class of medications known as anticonvulsants is used to treat and prevent seizures in patients with neurological diseases like epilepsy or other conditions. These medications stabilise the electrical activity in the brain, which lessens the frequency and intensity of seizures. Anticonvulsants can be categorised into a number of different groups, each of which has a unique method of action and a unique set of potential side effects.

A barbiturate called phenobarbital acts by increasing the impact of the inhibitory neurotransmitter GABA. It has been around for a while and is one of the most well-known anticonvulsants. It is frequently used with other anticonvulsants, although because of its long half-life, it only needs to be taken once or twice day. However, when using phenobarbital, some people, especially older adults, may develop negative side effects such fatigue, confusion, and other mental disorders.

Another often prescribed anticonvulsant drug is carbamazepine. This medicine decreases the excitability of neurons by inhibiting sodium channels in the brain. Partial seizures are one of the disorders that trigeminal neuralgia is highly effective in treating. It is a type of chronic pain. Contrarily, carbamazepine may have unfavourable symptoms like nausea and dizziness and may interact unfavourably with other medications.

Another anticonvulsant, valproic acid, decreases the excitatory neurotransmitter glutamate's activity while increasing that of the inhibitory neurotransmitter GABA. It is effective in treating a variety of seizure types, such as absence seizures and generalised seizures, and it can also be used to stave off migraines. Valproic acid, on the other hand, has occasionally been associated with a higher risk of adverse effects, including weight gain, hair loss, and liver damage.

The more recent anticonvulsants that have been produced include lamotrigine, topiramate, and levetiracetam. Topiramate works by raising the activity of GABA while decreasing the activity of glutamate, whilst lamotrigine works by reducing the quantity of glutamate released into the brain. Levetiracetam seems to work by binding to SV2A, a specific type of protein involved in controlling the release of neurotransmitters in the brain. Although modern medications are generally more well-tolerated and have fewer side effects than earlier anticonvulsants, some patients may still experience sleepiness, dizziness, and other symptoms.

Anticonvulsants may help people with epilepsy or other neurological conditions better control their seizures and experience a higher quality of life as a result. They should, however, be used with caution and under close observation because, if not, they could interfere with other medications and have major negative effects. Anticonvulsant users should keep their primary care physician informed of any unusual symptoms or side effects and keep that line of contact open.

Antiparkinson agents

Parkinson's disease is a neurological disorder that impairs movement in sufferers. Drugs called "antiparkinson agents" are used to treat Parkinson's disease. Parkinson's disease is brought on by the degeneration or destruction of particular dopamine-producing nerve cells in the brain. A neurotransmitter known as dopamine is crucial for controlling movement. Numerous symptoms, such as tremors, rigidity, slowness of movement, and issues with balance and coordination, are associated with Parkinson's disease. Although there is no cure for Parkinson's disease, antiparkinson medications can help people manage their symptoms and improve their quality of life.

Antiparkinson medications can be divided into a number of different classes, each of which has a distinct mechanism of action and set of side effects. The three main categories of psychoactive compounds are dopaminergic medicines, anticholinergic substances, and MAO-B inhibitors.

Dopaminergic agents are drugs that increase the brain's concentration of the dopamine neurotransmitter. Because levodopa can be converted into dopamine in the brain, it is the most commonly utilised dopaminergic substance. Levodopa is frequently given along with carbidopa, which prevents levodopa from being broken down in the bloodstream before it reaches the brain. Two other categories of dopaminergic medications include dopamine agonists and COMT inhibitors. While COMT inhibitors function by preventing the body from breaking down levodopa, dopamine agonists act by stimulating dopamine receptors in the brain.

The neurotransmitter acetylcholine, which is involved in the control of movement, is inhibited by a class of drugs known as anticholinergic drugs. Patients with Parkinson's disease who take these drugs might have fewer rigidity and tremors as a result. However, especially in elderly people, they have the potential to induce negative side effects such dry mouth, constipation, and confusion.

Drugs referred to as MAO-B inhibitors function by inhibiting the monoamine oxidase B enzyme, which is in charge of destroying dopamine in the brain. By blocking the enzyme that breaks down dopamine, MAO-B inhibitors are able to enhance motor function and raise dopamine levels in the brain. They are frequently used in conjunction with other drugs that treat Parkinson's disease.

Despite their potential efficacy in easing Parkinson's disease symptoms, antiparkinson medicines have a number of potential side effects. When taking dopaminergic drugs, common side responses include nausea, vomiting, and hallucinations. Constipation, dry mouth, and visual impairment are all potential side effects of anticholinergic drugs. Aside from headaches and nausea, adverse effects of MAO-B drugs could also include insomnia. Medical personnel must thoroughly evaluate their patients before prescribing antiparkinson medications, and they must continue to do so to spot any negative side effects.

In addition to medication therapy, alternative options for treating Parkinson's disease include deep brain stimulation, physical therapy, and speech therapy. Electrodes can be implanted in the brain as part of deep brain stimulation to help with movement control. Taking a holistic, multidisciplinary approach to patient treatment is frequently required in order to support patients in controlling their symptoms and maintaining their quality of life.

Antipsychotics

The symptoms of severe mental illnesses like schizophrenia, major depressive disorder, and bipolar disorder are treated with antipsychotics, a class of drugs. Neuroleptics, the other name for antipsychotics, are often used. By concentrating on specific brain neurotransmitters linked in the illness, such as dopamine and serotonin, these medications lessen the severity of symptoms.

There are two types of antipsychotic drugs: conventional and atypical. Typical antipsychotics were the first medications developed to treat psychosis. The term "first-generation antipsychotics" is also used to describe them. Second-generation antipsychotics, also known as atypical antipsychotics, are a more recent class of antipsychotic drugs that were created after typical antipsychotics and are linked to a lower risk of side effects.

As part of their mechanism of action, antipsychotic drugs inhibit the dopamine receptors in the brain. A neurotransmitter known as dopamine has been connected to sensations of pleasure, reward, and motivation. It is possible for persons with specific mental illnesses to produce an excessive quantity of dopamine, which can lead to symptoms including hallucinations, delusions, and disorganised thinking. By preventing dopamine receptors in the brain from functioning, antipsychotic medications can lower the severity of these symptoms.

Antipsychotics can be administered to a patient in a number various ways, the most popular of which being injections, oral pills, and long-acting formulations. The choice of which drug to take and how it should be administered depends on the patient's condition, medical history, and personal response to treatment.

Users of antipsychotic drugs typically report unpleasant side effects such sluggishness, weight gain, dry mouth, diarrhea, and blurred vision. Atypical antipsychotics have a better response from patients than traditional antipsychotics since they are linked to less side effects. On the other hand, atypical antipsychotics have been linked to a higher risk of metabolic side effects, including diabetes and high cholesterol.

To treat the symptoms of mental illness, antipsychotic drugs are routinely used in conjunction with other therapies. Social support and psychotherapy are potential treatments. Although they are not a cure for many conditions, they can help patients manage their symptoms and enhance the quality of their lives.

It is crucial to remember that antipsychotic medications should never be taken without a licenced medical professional's supervision and direction. These medications are known to have serious side effects, such as movement disorders like tardive dyskinesia, which can sometimes be permanent. Regular patient evaluations should check for the incidence of these side effects, and dosage adjustments should be made as needed.

Antipsychotics may also be ineffective for treating some medical conditions and may interfere badly with the effects of other medications, including those that are over-the-counter. Patients are advised to speak with their primary care physician about all current medications they are taking as well as any existing medical conditions before starting antipsychotic treatment.

A large class of medications called antipsychotics is used to treat and manage the signs and symptoms of severe mental illness. They achieve this by preventing the brain's dopamine receptors from functioning, which reduces the severity of symptoms including hallucinations, delusions, and distorted thinking. Antipsychotic users should maintain a close contact with their doctor in order to be closely monitored because these medications have potential negative effects. Antipsychotic drugs are routinely recommended along with other treatments in order to manage mental illness and improve the patient's quality of life.

Bipolar agents

Manic or hypomanic highs and depressive lows alternately occur during periods of the psychiatric disease known as bipolar disorder. It necessitates ongoing therapy because it is a chronic condition. Patients with bipolar disorder are usually prescribed members of the "bipolar agents" medication family. They achieve this by establishing a condition of mental balance and averting episodes of mania, hypomania, and depression. Bipolar drugs fall into a few different types, each with its own mode of action and distinct potential side effects.

Mood Stabilizers

The cornerstone of treatment for those with bipolar disorder is mood stabilisers. They are efficient because they lessen the intensity and frequency of manic episodes and stop depressive episodes from happening. The mood stabiliser with the oldest history and highest usage rate is lithium. It has been shown to help treat both manic and depressed episodes that may happen as a result of having bipolar disorder. On the other hand, it could result in negative side effects like weight gain, kidney damage, and hand tremors. Lamotrigine, carbamazepine, and valproate are other mood stabilisers.

Atypical Antipsychotics

Bipolar disorder has been successfully treated using atypical antipsychotics, a new class of antipsychotic medications. The 1990s were a decade of drug development. They work by specifically affecting the dopamine and serotonin receptors in the brain. They can be used alone or in combination with mood stabilisers to treat manic episodes. Patients with bipolar disorder are routinely prescribed atypical antipsychotic drugs such aripiprazole, quetiapine, olanzapine, and risperidone. These medications may have negative side effects such sleepiness and increased hunger in addition to raising the risk of diabetes and cardiovascular disease.

Antidepressants

Patients with bipolar disorder may be given antidepressants as a type of medication, especially during depressed episodes. On the other hand, they are also known to trigger manic episodes in some bipolar illness patients. As a result, these medications are frequently used along with a mood stabiliser or an antipsychotic in the treatment of manic episodes. Patients who have been given a bipolar illness diagnosis commonly get antidepressants such fluoxetine, sertraline, and bupropion. These medications have been related to a range of negative side effects, including nausea, sexual dysfunction, and weight gain.

Other Medications

Stimulants, which may be used to lessen the symptoms of depression, as well as benzodiazepines, which may be used to treat anxiety and sleeplessness, are other drugs that may be used to treat bipolar disorder. Lithium and valproic acid are two other drugs that may be used to treat bipolar illness. However, it is generally not advised that these medications be taken for an extended period of time due to the risk of addiction as well as other potential side effects.

Patients with bipolar disorder are usually prescribed members of the "bipolar agents" medication family. Mood stabilisers are the cornerstone of treatment, however atypical antipsychotics and antidepressants may also be used, depending on the specific symptoms being treated. Every drug has a different mechanism of action and a distinct set of potential side effects. When choosing a drug, it is important to examine the individual needs and bipolar disorder symptoms of the patient. Determining the medicine and dosage that will be most beneficial in treating bipolar disorder requires close collaboration with a medical specialist.

Antidepressants

A class of medications known as antidepressants is used to treat mood disorders such as depression, anxiety, and others. Antidepressants come in a variety of forms, such as tricyclic antidepressants (TCAs), selective serotonin reuptake inhibitors (SSRIs), serotonin-norepinephrine reuptake inhibitors (SNRIs), and monoamine oxidase inhibitors (MAOIs).

The most often prescribed antidepressants, SSRIs, function by raising serotonin levels in the brain. A chemical called serotonin controls mood, hunger, and sleep. Fluoxetine (Prozac), sertraline

(Zoloft), and citalopram (Celexa) are examples of popular SSRIs.

SNRIs function by raising the brain's levels of serotonin and norepinephrine. A neurotransmitter that controls arousal and mood is norepinephrine. Venlafaxine (Effexor) and duloxetine (Cymbalta) are examples of common SNRIs.

TCAs function by preventing the brain's reuptake of serotonin and norepinephrine. This enhances the brain's supply of these neurotransmitters. Amitriptyline (Elavil) and nortriptyline (Pamelor) are two popular TCAs.

MAOIs function by preventing the monoamine oxidase enzyme from degrading serotonin and norepinephrine in the brain. Phenelzine (Nardil) and tranylcypromine (Parnate) are examples of common MAOIs.

Antidepressants frequently cause nausea, dizziness, dry mouth, and sexual dysfunction as adverse effects. Suicidal thoughts or actions could be more severe adverse effects, particularly in kids, teenagers, and young adults.

Anxiolytics, sedatives and hypnotics

Antidepressants, a class of medication, are primarily used to treat severe depressive illness, anxiety disorders, and other mood disorders. They alter the amounts of particular neurotransmitters in the brain in order to have an effect. These neurotransmitters control hunger, sleep, and mood. They also contain serotonin, norepinephrine, and dopamine. Antidepressants can be divided into a number of different groups, each of which has a unique method of action and might be connected to a specific set of side effects.

The kind of antidepressants most usually prescribed to patients are selective serotonin reuptake inhibitors (SSRIs). They must particularly block the reuptake of serotonin, a neurotransmitter in the brain that regulates mood, in order to have their desired effects. Serotonin levels are increased as a result, which can improve mood and lower the severity of depression symptoms. Selected serotonin reuptake inhibitors include the antidepressants citalopram (Celexa), sertraline (Zoloft), and fluoxetine (Prozac).

Serotonin and norepinephrine reuptake inhibitors, or SNRIs for short, are another kind of antidepressant. The reason SNRIs work is because they stop the brain from reabsorbing serotonin and norepinephrine. In addition to easing the signs of anxiety and chronic pain, this may also improve mood. Examples of SNRIs include the antidepressants duloxetine (Cymbalta) and venlafaxine (Effexor).

Tricyclic antidepressants, or TCAs, are a more established type of antidepressants that work by preventing the brain's neurotransmitters like serotonin and norepinephrine from being reabsorbed. Despite the fact that they are effective in the treatment of depression, doctors prefer to give them far less frequently than they do other, more recent antidepressants due to the higher risk of more serious side effects. TCAs include amitriptyline (marketed under the name Elavil) and imipramine (marketed under the name Tofranil).

Monoamine oxidase inhibitors (MAOIs), which are antidepressants, work by blocking the monoamine oxidase enzyme, which breaks down neurotransmitters like serotonin, norepinephrine, and dopamine. One type of antidepressant is the MAOI. By inhibiting an enzyme that prevents these neurotransmitters from reaching their full capacity in the brain, MAOIs improve mood. MAOIs are effective antidepressants, but due to the potential for negative interactions with specific foods and medications, doctors choose to prescribe them less frequently than other forms of antidepressants. Two examples of MAOIs are phenelzine (marketed as Nardil) and tranylcypromine (marketed as Parnate).

Atypical antidepressants are a large category of antidepressants that function to elevate mood in a number of different ways. Typically, if a patient has tried other antidepressants and discovered that they were ineffective or had intolerable side effects, a doctor would recommend them. Atypical antidepressants include trazodone (marketed as Desyrel), mirtazapine (marketed as Remeron), and bupropion (marketed as Wellbutrin).

It is well known that antidepressants may have a multitude of side effects, some of which include gastrointestinal problems, vertigo, a dry mouth, weight gain, sexual dysfunction, and trouble sleeping. They can also make suicidal thoughts and actions more likely, especially in kids, teenagers, and young adults. This is especially true when other risk factors are included. Antidepressant-treated patients should be closely monitored for any negative side effects, such as behavioural or mood abnormalities. Antidepressants have the potential to trigger manic episodes, thus anyone with a history of bipolar disorder or a family history of the condition should use extreme caution when taking these drugs.

Antidepressants are a crucial part of the treatment for depression as well as other mood disorders. They have the potential to help improve a patient's mood and general quality of life when used properly and under the supervision of a skilled medical professional.

Cholinergies

Acetylcholine, a neurotransmitter in the nervous system, is stimulated or made more active by cholinergic medicines, commonly referred to as cholinergics. These medications are used to treat a number of ailments, such as urinary retention, glaucoma, myasthenia gravis, and Alzheimer's disease. The mechanisms of action, indications, side effects, and contraindications of cholinergic medications will all be covered in this article.

Mechanism of Action

A neurotransmitter called acetylcholine is essential for the movement of nerve impulses between neurons and muscle cells. In order to increase the levels of acetylcholine, cholinergic medicines stimulate the action of acetylcholine receptors in the neurological system. Numerous physiological responses result from this, such as an increase in heart rate, gastrointestinal motility, perspiration, and salivation.

Indications

Several conditions are treated with cholinergic medications, including:

Alzheimer's disease

Galantamine, donepezil, and rivastigmine are a few examples of cholinesterase inhibitors that are used to treat the cognitive signs and symptoms of Alzheimer's disease.

Myasthenia gravis

When myasthenia gravis causes muscle weakness, acetylcholinesterase inhibitors like neostigmine and pyridostigmine are used as a treatment.

Glaucoma

The increased intraocular pressure brought on by glaucoma is treated with cholinergic agonists like carbachol and pilocarpine.

Urinary retention

Bethanechol and other cholinergic agonists are used to promote bladder contractions and treat urine retention.

Side Effects

The physiological effects that cholinergic medications have on the body are connected to their adverse effects. These may consist of:

Nausea and vomiting

Cholinergic medications may cause nausea and vomiting by accelerating gastrointestinal motility.

Diarrhea

Drugs that promote gastrointestinal motility, such as cholinergics, can cause diarrhoea.

Sweating

Cholinergic medications may cause more sweating, which some patients may find uncomfortable.

Salivation

Cholinergic medications can make people salivate more, which some patients may find irritating.

Bradycardia

Drugs that are cholinergic can lower heart rate, which may be troublesome for those who already have bradycardia.

Hypotension

Cholinergic medications can lower blood pressure, which can be dangerous for those who already have hypotension.

Contraindications

Patients with: are contraindicated for cholinergic medications.

Hypersensitivity

Some patients may experience an allergic reaction from cholinergic medications.

Asthma

Drugs that are cholinergic can make asthma symptoms worse.

Peptic ulcer disease

Drugs that promote cholinergic activity may aggravate peptic ulcer disease by increasing stomach acid output.

Urinary obstruction

Drugs that block choline can make urinary blockage worse.

Bradycardia

Drugs that block choline can aggravate bradycardia that already exists.

A class of pharmaceuticals known as cholinergic drugs works to increase or promote the action of the neurotransmitter acetylcholine in the nervous system. These medications are used to treat a number of ailments, such as urinary retention, glaucoma, myasthenia gravis, and Alzheimer's disease. In individuals with specific medical disorders, cholinergic medicines should not be used due to their potential adverse effects, which are correlated with their physiological effects on the body. Cholinergic pharmaceuticals should be used under the guidance of a trained healthcare professional, as with other medications.

Anticholinergics

Anticholinergics are a class of medications that limit the action of the neurotransmitter acetylcholine. Acetylcholine is responsible for a variety of bodily functions, including the regulation of muscular contractions, mood, and cognitive processes. These medications are prescribed for the treatment of a wide variety of medical illnesses, such as urinary incontinence, digestive disorders, and respiratory infections. In this piece, we will go through the action mechanism, applications, potential adverse effects, and safety measures associated with anticholinergic medicines.

Mechanism of Action

By attaching to the receptors for acetylcholine in the central and peripheral nervous systems, anticholinergic medicines are able to inhibit the function of this neurotransmitter. Acetylcholine plays a role in the transmission of nerve impulses that are responsible for the regulation of a variety of activities, including the contraction of muscles, the pace of the heart, and digestion. Anticholinergic medicines work to diminish the activity of the parasympathetic nervous system by inhibiting the action of acetylcholine. The parasympathetic nervous system is the part of the nervous system that is responsible for relaxing the body and conserving energy. This brings about a number of effects, some of which include a reduction in secretions, relaxation of smooth muscles, and an acceleration of the heart rate.

Uses

Anticholinergic medications are utilized in the treatment of many illnesses, including the following:

Urinary incontinence

Anticholinergic medications, such as oxybutynin and tolterodine, are utilized in the treatment of urine incontinence. These medications work to treat the condition by reducing the number of bladder contractions and increasing the capacity of the bladder.

Gastrointestinal disorders

Anticholinergic medications, such as dicyclomine and hyoscyamine, are employed in the treatment of gastrointestinal conditions like irritable bowel syndrome (IBS) and peptic ulcers. These medications work to alleviate stomach and intestine spasms by inhibiting the activity of cholinergic receptors.

Respiratory diseases

By relaxing the smooth muscles of the airways, anticholinergic medications like ipratropium and tiotropium are used to treat respiratory ailments like chronic obstructive pulmonary disease (COPD) and asthma. These diseases are caused by inflammation of the airways.

Parkinson's disease

By inhibiting the activity of acetylcholine in the brain, Parkinson's disease symptoms like tremors and stiffness in the muscles can be treated using anticholinergic medications like benztropine and trihexyphenidyl. These medications work by relaxing the muscles and reducing the amount of acetylcholine in the brain.

Side Effects

Anticholinergic medications have been linked to a number of adverse effects, including the following:

Dry mouth

The production of saliva can be inhibited by anticholinergic medications, which can result in a dry mouth.

Constipation

The digestive process can be slowed down by anticholinergic medications, which can result in constipation.

Blurred vision

Vision can get blurry and it may be difficult to concentrate when taking anticholinergic medications.

Urinary retention

Anticholinergic medications have been shown to inhibit bladder contractions, which can make it difficult to urinate.

Confusion

Anticholinergic medicines have been shown to be able to permeate the blood-brain barrier and alter cognitive functioning, which can result in memory loss and disorientation.

Precautions

When treating people who have particular medical disorders, such as the following, anticholinergic medications have to be used with extreme caution:

Glaucoma

Anticholinergic medications have been shown to raise intraocular pressure, which can accelerate the progression of glaucoma.

Enlarged prostate

The symptoms of an enlarged prostate, such as having trouble peeing, might be made worse by the use of anticholinergic medications.

Cardiovascular disease

Patients who have cardiovascular illness are more likely to experience an increased heart rate and arrhythmias if they use anticholinergic medications.

Kidney and liver disease

Patients who suffer from conditions affecting either the kidneys or the liver should have their use of anticholinergic medicines closely monitored. These organs are responsible for the drug's elimination from the body.

Anticholinergic pharmaceuticals are a class of medications that limit the activity of acetylcholine. These medications are utilized in the treatment of a wide variety of ailments, including urinary incontinence, gastrointestinal disorders, and respiratory diseases. On the other hand, using anticholinergic medication can cause a wide variety of adverse effects, such as dry mouth, constipation, impaired vision, forgetfulness, and memory impairment. To reduce the likelihood of unpleasant side effects, it is vital to use anticholinergic medications with extreme caution and only after consulting a qualified medical professional.

Adrenergies

Medications of the adrenergic class are used to treat issues with the sympathetic nervous system. Norepinephrine and epinephrine, also known as adrenaline, are two hormones that are mimicked by these treatments. Conditions as diverse as asthma, heart failure, shock, and excessive blood pressure are all managed with these drugs. Adrenergic pharmaceuticals are also known as sympathomimetic medicines due to their ability to mimic the effects of the sympathetic nervous system.

The adrenergic drug classification system is broken down into two main categories: direct-acting and indirect-acting. Some adrenergic medications have an indirect effect by preventing the body from reabsorbing norepinephrine or by raising the quantity of norepinephrine produced from nerve endings. Drugs that affect on the adrenergic system directly target the receptors themselves.

Drugs that act on the adrenergic system directly include:

Epinephrine

The hormone and neurotransmitter epinephrine is produced by the adrenal gland. As a potent stimulator of alpha and beta adrenergic receptors, it is used to treat life-threatening allergic responses, asthma, and cardiac arrest.

Norepinephrine

The neurotransmitter norepinephrine is secreted by sympathetic nervous system neurons. This medicine is an effective alpha-adrenergic receptor activator, making it useful for the treatment of shock and hypotension.

Phenylephrine

In addition to its role as a decongestant, phenylephrine is used to treat hypotension because it is a selective alpha-1 adrenergic receptor agonist.

Dopamine

Dopamine is a precursor to norepinephrine and functions as a neurotransmitter that interacts with dopamine receptors. The brain and spinal cord both contain dopamine receptors. It is useful in treating a variety of medical emergencies, including shock and heart failure.

These drugs have indirect adrenergic effects and are examples:

Amphetamines

An amphetamine's effect on the CNS makes it a stimulant. The amount of norepinephrine and dopamine released from nerve terminals is increased due to these medicines. These drugs are effective in the treatment of attention deficit hyperactivity disorder (ADHD) as well as narcolepsy.

Cocaine

Cocaine can be used as a local anesthetic, but it also blocks norepinephrine reuptake effectively.

Monoamine oxidase inhibitors (MAOIs)

Norepinephrine and other brain chemicals are protected from breakdown by monoamine oxidase inhibitors (MAOIs). Patients with Parkinson's disease and major depression are often prescribed them.

Tricyclic antidepressants (TCAs)

TCA-class antidepressants block the brain's ability to recycle certain neurotransmitters, including norepinephrine and others. Anxiety, sadness, and neuropathic pain are all treated with them.

While adrenergic medicines have useful therapeutic applications, they can also have significant negative side effects. The most common unwanted effects of adrenergic drugs include tremors, a quicker heart rate, and higher blood pressure. Anxiety is another side effect of adrenergic medicines. Adrenergic drugs may cause unwanted effects like anxiety, insomnia, and headaches.

Adrenergic medicines should be used with considerable caution when treating patients with cardiovascular disease, hypertension, or hyperthyroidism. These medications should be used with caution in patients who are also taking other medications that increase blood pressure or heart rate, such as decongestants or weight loss medications.

Medications of the adrenergic class are used to treat issues with the sympathetic nervous system. These medicines mimic the hormones norepinephrine and epinephrine to alleviate symptoms. They are used to treat a variety of conditions, the most prevalent of which being asthma, heart failure, shock, and high blood pressure. Adrenergic drugs should be used with caution in some patient populations due to the potential for severe side effects. Medical providers should carefully weigh the benefits and risks of adrenergic medicines before prescribing them to patients.

Adrenergic antagonists

Norepinephrine is a neurotransmitter in the sympathetic nervous system, and its function can be blocked with a class of pharmaceuticals called adrenergic antagonists. Hypertension, heart failure, and some forms of arrhythmia are just some of the problems that these medications are used to treat. Adrenergic antagonists inhibit the effects of norepinephrine by binding to and inhibiting alpha and beta receptors. As a result, the smooth muscle in the airways and blood arteries relaxes, the heart rate slows, and the blood pressure drops.

Adrenergic antagonists fall into several distinct categories, each with its own mode of action and clinical uses. Among these are the alpha-, beta-, and combined alpha-beta-blockers.

To counteract the effects of norepinephrine on alpha receptors, doctors use alpha blockers, also called alpha-adrenergic antagonists. This makes alpha blockers beneficial for treating hypertension, benign prostatic hyperplasia (BPH), and other diseases involving urine retention as they stimulate blood vessel dilatation and smooth muscle relaxation in the bladder and prostate gland. The alpha blockers doxazosin, prazosin, and terazosin are all good examples.

Beta-adrenergic antagonists, often known as beta blockers, prevent norepinephrine from activating beta receptors. Based on their specificity for beta-1 or beta-2 receptors, beta blockers can be further subdivided into three types. Angina, arrhythmias, and hypertension are treated with nonselective beta blockers, while beta-1 selective blockers are used largely for these conditions. As a result of its ability to generate bronchoconstriction, beta-2 selective blockers are largely utilized in the treatment of asthma and chronic obstructive pulmonary disease (COPD). Beta blockers are used to reduce heart rate and blood pressure.

Mixed alpha-beta blockers, or alpha-beta blockers, prevent norepinephrine from binding to its alpha and beta receptors. As a result, the smooth muscle in the airways and blood arteries relaxes, the heart rate slows, and the blood pressure drops. Treatments for high blood pressure and heart failure frequently use alpha-beta blockers. Carvedilol and labetalol are two common alpha-beta blockers.

Fatigue, dizziness, hypotension, and erectile dysfunction are all possible side effects of adrenergic antagonists. Rebound hypertension, angina, and arrhythmias are only some of the complications that might result from suddenly stopping beta blockers. Adrenergic antagonist patients should be continuously monitored for these adverse effects and advised against suddenly stopping treatment.

Certain medical disorders, such as severe hypotension, bradycardia, heart block, asthma, and chronic obstructive pulmonary disease (COPD), rule out the use of adrenergic antagonists. Patients with diabetes should exercise caution when using them because they can hide the signs of hypoglycemia.

Medications known as adrenergic antagonists prevent alpha and beta receptors from responding to norepinephrine. Hypertension, heart failure, and some forms of arrhythmia are only some of the problems they are used to treat. Patients taking adrenergic antagonists should be carefully watched for unwanted effects, as they can occur. Patients with specific medical disorders, such as diabetes, are advised against taking them. Adrenergic antagonists, like any other medicine, should not be taken without first discussing them with a doctor.

Hypothalamic and pituitary drugs

Pharmaceuticals that act on the hypothalamus and pituitary gland to control hormone release are known collectively as "hypothalamic and pituitary" drugs. Many different medical problems are treated with these medications. Hormonal abnormalities, infertility, growth issues, and even some types of cancer are just some of the many conditions for which these drugs are recommended.

Reproductive health issues can be treated using drugs that target the hypothalamus and pituitary gland, such as gonadotropin-releasing hormone (GnRH) agonists. They are also among the most often utilized medications today. GnRH agonists are effective in the treatment of a wide variety of conditions, including endometriosis, prostate cancer, and uterine fibroids. These drugs are effective because they reduce the amount of estrogen and testosterone your body makes. Hormones that act as GnRH agonists include leuprolide, nafarelin, and goserelin.

Another class of drugs that can affect the hypothalamus and pituitary glands are called dopamine agonists. By interacting with dopamine receptors in the brain, these medications stimulate the production of the feel-good chemical. Patients with conditions like restless legs syndrome, pituitary tumors, and Parkinson's disease are given these drugs. Dopamine receptor agonists include drugs like pramipexole, ropinirole, and cabergoline.

Somatostatin analogs are another class of drugs used to treat hormonal disorders, especially those related to growth hormone (GH). Somatostatin analogs are a class of drugs employed in the management of acromegaly and gigantism. Growth hormone (GH) and other hormone synthesis is inhibited by these drugs. Octreotide and lanreotide are two examples of somatostatin analogs.

In addition to these classes of drugs, there are others that can modify the hypothalamus' and pituitary gland's production of specific hormones. The hypothalamus secretes oxytocin, a hormone involved in a wide range of physiological activities. These include the contractions of the uterus during delivery and the regulation of social behavior. Synthetic oxytocin has several medicinal applications, including inducing labor and promoting lactation in nursing mothers. It is also used to treat conditions such as autism and anxiety.

Vasopressin, also called antidiuretic hormone, is a hormone generated by the brain that helps regulate the body's water balance. Many medical conditions, such as diabetes insipidus, nocturnal enuresis, and bleeding disorders, are managed using desmopressin or another synthetic vasopressin.

There is a wide range of potential side effects associated with medications that act on the hypothalamus and pituitary gland. Common negative responses include sickness, vomiting, headache, and fatigue. Long-term usage of these drugs may increase the risk of major side effects such low bone density, diabetes, and heart disease.

Hormonal disorders and growth issues, among others, are treated with medications of the hypothalamus and pituitary drug class. These drugs achieve their therapeutic effects by controlling hormone production via acting on the hypothalamus and pituitary gland. These drugs may be useful in the treatment of a wide range of illnesses, but they also carry the risk of serious side effects and should be taken only when absolutely necessary and under the care of a medical expert.

Thyroid and antithyroid drugs

Thyroid issues like hypothyroidism, hyperthyroidism, and goiter are treated with thyroid and antithyroid medicines. These medications are designed to either increase or decrease the body's natural production of thyroid hormones. Growth and development, as well as metabolic regulation, rely heavily on thyroid hormones.

Thyroid Hormones

The thyroid gland is responsible for secreting two major hormones, thyroxine (or T4) and triiodothyronine (or T3). The rate at which the body's cells digest food is regulated by these hormones. A wide variety of other organs rely on them for their development and function as well, including the brain, heart, and digestive system.

Hypothyroidism

Hypothyroidism is a condition in which the thyroid gland does not produce enough of the hormones needed to control thyroid activity. Fatigue, weight gain, aversion to cold, and constipation are just some of the symptoms that might arise from this. The most commonly prescribed treatment for hypothyroidism is levothyroxine (Synthroid), a synthetic version of the T4 hormone. Levothyroxine should only be used orally once a day. Dosage adjustments are often made based on the patient's symptoms and thyroid hormone levels.

Hyperthyroidism

Hyperthyroidism is characterized by the thyroid gland's excessive synthesis of thyroid hormone. Some of the possible outcomes of this condition are decreased appetite, tremors, anxiety, and heat intolerance. Several treatments, including antithyroid drugs and radioactive iodine, are available to treat the medical condition known as hyperthyroidism.

Antithyroid Drugs

Hyperthyroidism can be effectively treated with antithyroid drugs since they work by reducing the body's synthesis of thyroid hormones. The most commonly used antithyroid medicine is methimazole, also known as Tapazole. Methimazole works by inhibiting an enzyme required for the synthesis of thyroid hormones. Another antithyroid medicine, propylthiouracil (PTU), has a higher risk of side effects than other antithyroid medications, hence it is used much less frequently. All of these drugs must be taken orally, and the typical course of treatment lasts anything from six months to two years.

Radioactive Iodine

Radioactive iodine therapy is being studied as a possible treatment for hyperthyroidism. The thyroid gland takes in very small amounts of radioactive iodine that are then analyzed. As a result of the radiation's destruction of thyroid tissue, less of these hormones are produced. Approximately 80% of patients see improvement with this medication, and it is often used when antithyroid drugs fail to do so or are uncomfortable.

Thyroid Cancer

Thyroid hormones are effective not just in treating thyroid disorders, but also in treating a variety of conditions, including thyroid cancer. Thyroid cancer treatment typically consists of surgical excision of the thyroid gland, followed by radioactive iodine therapy to eradicate any remaining cancer cells. Thyroid hormone replacement treatment (THRT) is a method used to restore hormone levels after surgical removal of the thyroid.

Side Effects

Thyroid and antithyroid drugs can cause a wide variety of side effects, including but not limited to headaches, nausea, diarrhea, and skin rashes. Rare but possible side effects of these drugs include liver damage, suppression of bone marrow production, and allergic reactions. Patients using these drugs who experience any unusual symptoms should contact their doctor immediately.

Thyroid and antithyroid medication are two essential drugs for treating thyroid disorders. These drugs influence the body's natural synthesis of thyroid hormones, increasing or decreasing their effect. Some people may experience negative consequences from using them, despite the fact that they are normally safe and effective. Patients who have been prescribed these drugs should be closely monitored by their doctor to ensure they are taking the prescribed amount and to detect any unwanted side effects early on.

Gonadal hormones and blockers

Gonadal hormones and blockers are a family of drugs used to alter the synthesis of sex hormones such as estrogen, progesterone, and testosterone. The effects of these hormones can also be blocked by these medications. In both sexes, these hormones play a crucial role in the development and maintenance of sexual traits and reproductive capacities. That holds true for both the development and upkeep of sexual traits as well as for reproductive processes.

The gonadal hormones and blockers can be categorized into the following groups:

Estrogen hormones

In addition to controlling the menstrual cycle and other secondary sexual characteristics in females, the female sex hormone estrogen is also crucial in the development of breast tissue and other female anatomical features. Secondary sexual characteristics may also be influenced by estrogen. Estrogen hormones have multiple medical applications, including HRT for postmenopausal women, cancer chemotherapy, and endometriosis treatment. One of the most widespread uses of estrogen hormones is in HRT.

Progesterone hormones

Progesterone, another female sex hormone, is mostly in charge of controlling the menstrual cycle and getting the uterus ready for conception. A common nickname for progesterone is "pregnancy hormone." Clinical uses of progesterone hormones include hormone replacement therapy (HRT) for postmenopausal women and the management of certain gynecological disorders.

Androgen hormones

Androgens, of which testosterone is one example, play a significant role in the maturation of males' tertiary sexual features, such as the expansion of facial hair and the deepening of the voice. A deeper voice is another characteristic that might emerge over time. The therapy of male hypogonadism and a subset of breast cancer are only two of the many medical uses for androgen hormones.

Gonadotropin-releasing hormone (GnRH) agonists and antagonists

Follicle-stimulating hormone (FSH) and luteinizing hormone (LH) production can be boosted by another hormone called gonadotropin-releasing hormone (GnRH). The synthesis of sex hormones in both sexes is controlled by the hormones follicle-stimulating hormone (FSH) and luteinizing hormone (LH). These hormones' production can be boosted by GnRH, a hormone that does the same. Both agonists and antagonists of the gonadotropin-releasing hormone (GnRH) are used in medicine for various purposes.

Selective estrogen receptor modulators (SERMs)

Selective estrogen receptor modulators are a group of drugs used to reduce estrogen's negative effects on various bodily systems. Clinical uses of SERMs include breast cancer prevention and treatment, as well as osteoporosis. SERMs are also used for the purpose of warding against and treating osteopenia.

Aromatase inhibitors

Aromatase is an enzyme that catalyzes the conversion of androgens to estrogens. Medications known as aromatase inhibitors block the enzyme responsible for estrogen production, hence lowering estrogen levels in the body. Aromatase inhibitors are a highly effective treatment for postmenopausal women with estrogen-dependent breast cancer.

Antiandrogens

To counteract the negative effects of androgens like testosterone on certain tissues, a family of drugs known as "antiandrogens" has been developed. The prostate, breast, and testicles are examples of such organs. Medication known as antiandrogens is used to treat conditions brought on by high levels of the male hormone androgen. Excessive hair growth (hirsutism) and prostate cancer are two instances.

These drugs require constant medical supervision due to the wide range of side effects they can produce and the potential drug interactions they can have. Pharmaceuticals that include gonadal hormones and blockers are included below. It's crucial to have an open dialogue with patients regarding the potential side effects of these medications on their fertility and sexual function before starting treatment.

Antidiabetic drugs and insulins

Increased blood glucose levels due to an inability to produce or properly use insulin characterize the chronic condition known as diabetes mellitus. To control and treat diabetes mellitus, doctors prescribe antidiabetic drugs and insulin. The long-term complications of diabetes, such as kidney failure, blindness, nerve damage, and cardiovascular disease, can be prevented by antidiabetic medication, which maintains blood glucose levels within the normal range.

Different classes of anti-diabetic drugs and insulins reduce blood glucose levels in slightly different ways. Which treatment choice is appropriate depends on the type of diabetes, the severity of the condition, and the patient's individual needs and preferences.

Biguanides

Biguanides, a class of oral diabetic treatments that includes the drug metformin, decrease glucose production in the liver while increasing insulin sensitivity in muscle and fat tissue. They do not result in hypoglycemia and do not promote insulin secretion. If you have type 2 diabetes, your doctor will likely prescribe metformin. In addition, it is often used in combination with other diabetes drugs.

Sulfonylureas

Sulfonylureas, such as glipizide and glyburide, are antidiabetic medicines because they stimulate insulin secretion by beta cells in the pancreas and are therefore used orally to treat diabetes. When metformin fails to control a person's type 2 diabetes, they are generally the next treatment option. They cause weight gain and raise the danger of hypoglycemia.

Meglitinides

Meglitinides, a class of oral diabetes drugs that includes repaglinide and nateglinide, work in a similar way to sulfonylureas by stimulating insulin synthesis in the pancreas, but their effects wear off more quickly. In addition to potentially causing hypoglycemia and weight gain, they are often administered in conjunction with a number of other diabetes drugs.

Alpha-glucosidase inhibitors

Alpha-glucosidase inhibitors, a class of oral antidiabetic drugs that includes the drugs acarbose and miglitol, work by delaying the digestion of carbohydrates and, by extension, the absorption of glucose in the small intestine. They do not result in hypoglycemia and do not promote insulin secretion. The majority of people with type 2 diabetes use them as a secondary treatment.

Thiazolidinediones

Thiazolidinediones are a class of oral diabetic medicines that boost insulin sensitivity in muscle and adipose tissue while decreasing glucose production in the liver. These drugs are usually only used as a second or third line of defense against type 2 diabetes because of the risks of weight gain, fluid retention, and heart failure.

Dipeptidyl peptidase-4 inhibitors

Sitagliptin and saxagliptin are two examples of dipeptidyl peptidase-4 inhibitors, a class of oral antidiabetic medications that increase insulin secretion from the pancreas while decreasing glucagon secretion. They are safe to use without fear of hypoglycemia and are often used as an adjunct treatment for type 2 diabetes.

Sodium-glucose cotransporter-2 inhibitors

Medications for diabetes like canagliflozin and dapagliflozin, which are sodium-glucose cotransporter-2 inhibitors, work by preventing the kidneys from reabsorbing glucose and increasing the amount of glucose that is expelled in urine. In addition, they raise insulin sensitivity in both muscle and fat tissue and reduce glucose production in the liver. They should only be used as a last resort because of the increased risk of amputations of the lower limbs and the possibility of inducing infections of the vaginal and urinary systems.

Insulins

Insulins are an injectable form of the antidiabetic medicine glyburide, which is used to supplement or replace the body's natural insulin in people with diabetes. The pancreas secretes the hormone insulin. Its principal role is to regulate blood sugar levels by facilitating glucose uptake and storage by cells. Diabetes, which is characterized by reduced insulin synthesis or activity, causes elevated blood glucose levels. The major objective of insulin therapy is to prevent diabetes-related complications such cardiovascular disease, neuropathy, and retinopathy.

Rapid-acting insulin, short-acting insulin, intermediate-acting insulin, and long-acting insulin are the most frequent types of insulin. Each patient's activity level, blood glucose levels, and meal pattern are taken into account while deciding which type of insulin to administer. A syringe, insulin pen, or insulin pump can all be used to administer insulin subcutaneously. Oral administration of insulin is possible.

Rapid-acting insulins are insulin analogs that have a fast onset of action (such as insulin lispro, insulin aspart, and insulin glulisine) but wear off quickly (often within 4 hours). These insulins are most effective when given before meals to prevent a sudden increase in blood sugar levels after eating. Rapid-acting insulins can also be delivered as a bolus dosage with an insulin pump to mimic the body's natural release of insulin in response to meal consumption.

Short-acting insulin, often known as "normal" insulin, can take up to 60 minutes to begin working and anywhere from 6 to 8 hours to completely wear off. It's taken before meals so that blood sugar doesn't surge afterward. Nonprescription insulin can be given using an insulin pump in the same way as basal and bolus doses are.

The effects of intermediate-acting insulins like NPH insulin don't kick in for the full 12–24 hours after they've been administered, but they do kick in within the first couple of hours. It is used to meet the needs for basal insulin before bed and between meals.

Long-acting insulin analogs, such insulin glargine and insulin detemir, have a slower onset of action but can last for up to 24 hours. In conjunction with rapid-acting or short-acting insulin, these are taken around-the-clock to cover glucose levels before, during, and after meals.

Anti-asthmatic drugs and drugs for COPD

Medication is available for a variety of respiratory conditions, including asthma and chronic obstructive pulmonary disease (COPD). These drugs work by lowering inflammation, soothing smooth muscle in the airways, and stopping bronchospasm from occurring. Asthma and chronic obstructive pulmonary disease (COPD) can be treated with a variety of medications, including bronchodilators, corticosteroids, leukotriene modifiers, and monoclonal antibodies.

In order to facilitate breathing, bronchodilators relax the airway's smooth muscle. Beta-agonists and anticholinergics are the two classes of bronchodilators. The beta-receptors in the lungs are targeted by the beta-agonists, which then relax the muscles surrounding the airways. Albuterol is a short-acting inhaler used in emergency situations, whereas salmeterol and formoterol are long-acting inhalers prescribed for maintenance treatment. Anticholinergics prevent the contraction of airway muscles by inhibiting the release of acetylcholine, a neurotransmitter. They can have a quick effect, like ipratropium, or a prolonged one, like tiotropium.

Inflammation in the airways can be reduced with the help of corticosteroids. The production of cytokines and other inflammatory mediators is suppressed, allowing them to function. It is possible to take corticosteroids orally, with an inhaler, or with a nebulizer. The most frequent type of corticosteroid used to treat asthma and COPD is the inhaled variety, which includes drugs like fluticasone and budesonide. Maintenance treatment employs them to lessen the occurrence and impact of symptoms. Exacerbations of chronic obstructive pulmonary disease (COPD) and asthma are treated temporarily with oral corticosteroids.

Inflammatory chemicals called leukotrienes are released during an asthma or COPD exacerbation, and leukotriene modifiers prevent their harmful effects. Inhaled corticosteroids have an alternative in leukotriene modifiers. They can be taken orally, like montelukast, or inhaled, as zafirlukast.

These severe forms of asthma and COPD are amenable to a newer family of medications called monoclonal antibodies. The inflammatory mediators in asthma and COPD are the targets of these biologic medicines. Omalizumab, mepolizumab, and dupilumab are all examples of monoclonal antibodies used to treat asthma. Roflumilast and benralizumab are two examples of monoclonal antibodies used to treat COPD.

These drugs are just one part of the overall treatment plan for asthma and COPD. Patients with severe COPD may benefit from oxygen therapy to raise their oxygen saturation levels. Patients with chronic obstructive pulmonary disease (COPD) can benefit from pulmonary rehabilitation, which consists of several activities such as exercise, breathing training, and education.

When choosing a treatment plan for asthma or COPD, healthcare providers must take into account the patient's medical history, present symptoms, and drug regimen. In addition to regular monitoring for symptom control and side effects, patients with asthma or COPD should be informed on the safe use of their medications. Asthma and chronic obstructive pulmonary disease patients who receive proper care can enjoy full, normal lives.

Drugs for peptic ulcer

Peptic ulcers are pathological conditions characterized by the development of open lesions within the mucosal lining of either the stomach or the small intestine. The most common causes of peptic ulcers are the bacteria Helicobacter pylori and the long-term use of nonsteroidal anti-inflammatory drugs (NSAIDs). Peptic ulcers are a painful condition. Symptoms of peptic ulcers include abdominal pain, nausea, vomiting, vomiting up blood, bloating, and loss of appetite. The infection caused by H. pylori can be treated with antibiotics, the production of stomach acid can be reduced with proton pump inhibitors (PPIs) or histamine-2 (H2) receptor antagonists, and the stomach lining can be protected with cytoprotective medications.

Antibiotics

Antibiotics are effective against H. pylori infections, the causative agent of peptic ulcer disease. Commonly used drugs include antibiotics including amoxicillin, clarithromycin, metronidazole, and tetracycline. Antibiotics work because they kill the bacteria or other microorganisms that are causing the ulcer's infection. Medications like proton pump inhibitors (PPIs) and H2 receptor antagonists are often prescribed alongside antibiotics for optimal results.

Proton Pump Inhibitors (PPIs)

Proton pump inhibitors (PPIs) are the go-to medication for peptic ulcer treatment. The drugs function by decreasing the production of stomach acid, which in turn reduces ulcer symptoms and promotes the body's natural ability to recover. Regularly prescribed proton pump inhibitors (PPIs) include omeprazole, lansoprazole, esomeprazole, pantoprazole, and rabeprazole. Oral dosing for four to eight weeks normally entails taking the medicine once day, 30 minutes before meals.

Histamine-2 (H2) Receptor Antagonists

Medication known as an H2 receptor antagonist is used to reduce gastric acid production by blocking the action of the histamine receptors. Because of this, fewer acids are generated. Peptic ulcer symptoms can be alleviated and the body's healing process sped up with the help of these drugs. Some common H2 receptor antagonists are cimetidine, ranitidine, famotidine, and nizatidine. The drugs are typically taken orally twice day, either before or after a meal, for a total of four to eight weeks.

Cytoprotective Agents

Stomach acid can cause serious damage to the stomach lining, but cytoprotective medicines can help protect it. The drugs are administered to speed up the ulcer's recovery and reduce the risk of complications like bleeding. Cytoprotective drugs such as sucralfate, misoprostol, and bismuth subsalicylate are often used. The medicine sucralfate helps the body create a barrier that keeps bacteria out of the ulcer. Medicines that reduce stomach acid production and promote healing include misoprostol and bismuth subsalicylate. The drugs are typically taken orally four to eight weeks prior to the start of each cycle, before each meal and before bed.

Mucosal Protective Agents

Mucosal protective agents are medicines that help an ulcer heal more quickly and reduce the risk of complications, such as bleeding, for the patient. Commonly used mucosal protective agents include carbenoxolone and rebamipide. Carbenoxolone is used to boost the stomach's natural defensive mechanism, while rebamipide is used to increase mucus production, both of which serve to protect the stomach lining. The effects of both of these drugs are enhanced when taken together. The drugs are typically taken orally four to eight weeks prior to the start of each cycle, before each meal and before bed.

Laxatives

Laxatives are drugs used to promote bowel movement frequency in those who suffer from constipation or other gastrointestinal problems. They work by stimulating intestinal activity or softening feces, both of which facilitate elimination. Depending on how they work, laxatives can be classified as stool softeners, osmotic laxatives, bulk-forming agents, or stimulant laxatives.

Emollient laxatives, often known as feces softeners, work by adding water to the feces, making it softer and easier to pass. This softens the experience of using the toilet. Sodium docusate is commonly used as a stool softener. Because of its lubricating properties, it is an effective treatment for constipation, whether administered orally or rectally.

Osmotic laxatives are effective because they attract water into the digestive system lumen, which stimulates bowel movement and softens feces. You can classify osmotic laxatives as either salt-containing or salt-free. Examples of saline laxatives include magnesium hydroxide, magnesium citrate, and sodium phosphate; examples of non-saline laxatives include lactulose, polyethylene glycol, and sorbitol.

Fiber supplements and other bulk-forming chemicals work to encourage bowel motions by increasing stool volume and water content. They are widely used for long-term use in the management of persistent constipation. Substances like psyllium and methylcellulose can be utilized to achieve this.

Stimulant laxatives cause bowel contractions because they cause muscular activity in the intestines. Because of this, bowel motility improves, leading to a higher frequency of bowel motions. Constipation is a common problem, so they are often used to alleviate that for a little while. Stimulating laxatives include bisacodyl and senna, among others.

Remember that laxative abuse can cause dependence, electrolyte imbalances, dehydration, and other serious side effects if used frequently or in large doses. Therefore, laxatives should only be used under the guidance of a medical practitioner for the short-term treatment of persistent constipation, and not as a long-term solution.

Combination laxatives are yet another category of laxatives that can be used in addition to the previously mentioned varieties. These laxatives are unique since they contain elements of more than one laxative. Some laxatives, for instance, combine the effects of a stool softener and a stimulant laxative into a single pill. Constipation can be managed with either bulk or liquid laxatives, however some people find that combination laxatives are more helpful than either on their own.

Laxatives are an effective therapeutic option for a variety of gastrointestinal issues, including constipation. However, its implementation must be carefully managed to avoid unwanted consequences and maximize their usefulness. In order to receive recommendations for the most effective treatment options, people with chronic constipation or other gastrointestinal disorders should discuss their symptoms with their primary care physician.

Antidiarrheals

Acute and chronic diarrhea, characterized by frequent, loose or watery bowel movements, can be treated well with antidiarrheal medications. Both acute and chronic diarrhea can be treated with antidiarrheal medication. Diarrhea can be caused by anything from an infection or inflammatory bowel disease to a food allergy or a reaction to a medicine. Antidiarrheal drugs reduce intestinal inflammation, cut down the frequency of bowel movements, and absorb extra fluids and electrolytes from the gut. In the following paragraphs, we will discuss the many types of antidiarrheal drugs and their mechanisms of action.

Opioid Antidiarrheals

Opioid antidiarrheals, such as loperamide (Imodium) and diphenoxylate with atropine (Lomotil), slow the digestive process and lengthen the duration between bowel movements. When taken orally, these medications slow down the digestive process, allowing for more fluid absorption. You can treat mild to moderate diarrhea with an over-the-counter drug called loperamide. Opioid diphenoxylate and anticholinergic atropine are used to treat gastrointestinal spasms, respectively. However, Lomotil, a medicine available only with a doctor's prescription, has both of these elements. Lomotil requires a prescription from your doctor.

Bismuth Subsalicylate

Pepto-Bismol, or bismuth subsalicylate, is a medication that can relieve diarrhea and reduce inflammation. This treatment works by coating the intestinal lining, which decreases inflammation and slows down bowel motions. Bismuth subsalicylate can reduce the severity and duration of diarrhea by neutralizing bacterial toxins in the intestines. This over-the-counter drug is widely used to alleviate the symptoms of diarrhea, both mild and severe, as well as stomach pain, heartburn, and indigestion.

Adsorbent Antidiarrheals

Absorbent antidiarrheals like kaolin and pectin (Kaopectate) work by preventing the absorption of toxins and other irritants in the digestive tract by adhering to them in the stomach. These remedies help the body absorb additional fluids and electrolytes, and they also lessen the frequency and severity of diarrhea. Kaolin and pectin, both of which may be purchased without a doctor's prescription, are common over-the-counter remedies for diarrhea of a mild to moderate severity.

Probiotics

Probiotics, or ingested living microorganisms, are effective at reestablishing the gut's normal bacterial composition and function. These microorganisms may aid in lowering inflammation, reestablishing regular bowel movements, and stopping the spread of harmful bacteria in the gut. Probiotics can be taken in a wide variety of forms, including pills, powders, and even yogurt. Many people take use of probiotic bacteria, such as Lactobacillus acidophilus, Bifidobacterium bifidum, and Saccharomyces boulardii.

Antisecretory Antidiarrheals

Antisecretory antidiarrheals, including racecadotril (Hidrasec), work by reducing the secretion of fluids and electrolytes in the stomach. These medications lessen the duration and intensity of diarrhea. Racecadotril is a medicine used to treat severe diarrhea in both adults and children. It is only available with a doctor's prescription. There is evidence that this medication can reduce the severity and duration of diarrhea, as well as avoid dehydration and electrolyte abnormalities. It has also been proven that this medicine lessens the possibility of electrolyte abnormalities occurring.

Antidiarrheal medications are a class of drugs used for the treatment and management of diarrhea. These drugs work by lowering inflammation, slowing the frequency of bowel movements, and soaking up extra fluids and electrolytes in the digestive tract.

Antibiotics that inhibit the synthesis of cell walls

Antibiotics are a class of drugs used to treat infections caused by bacteria. Antibiotics come in a wide variety of classes, each of which targets a particular bacterial cell component. One class of drugs known to inhibit cellular wall synthesis is the beta-lactam antibiotics.

Beta-lactams are a class of antibiotics that includes penicillin, monobactams, cephalosporins, and carbapenems, among others. These antibiotics are effective because they stop the bacteria from making the cell wall they need to survive in nature. The bacterial cell wall is composed of a complex polymer called peptidoglycan. Its principal role is to supply structural support for the cell. The beta-lactam class of antibiotics targets enzymes involved in peptidoglycan biosynthesis. This prevents the bacterial cell from constructing a protective cell wall, which leads to the bacteria's demise.

The penicillin family of beta-lactam antibiotics has been around the longest and is widely used today. Some gram-negative bacteria can also be killed by these antibiotics, which complements their effectiveness against gram-positive bacteria. Penicillin's beta-lactam ring is responsible for the antibiotic's antibacterial effects. Penicillins are classified into several groups based on their activity spectrum and their resistance to bacterial enzymes that break down the beta-lactam ring.

A class of antibiotics known as cephalosporins, cephalosporins are structurally similar to penicillins but are effective against gram-positive and gram-negative bacteria. Physically, penicillins and cephalosporins are very similar, but cephalosporins are the more potent antibiotic. All cephalosporins, like penicillins, have a beta-lactam ring, however unlike penicillins, cephalosporins are more resistant to the bacterial enzymes that destroy this ring, making them more effective against some bacteria. Cephalosporin generations are primarily determined by two factors: the breadth of cephalosporins' activities and their resistance to bacterial enzymes.

Monobactam antibiotics are easily identifiable by their unique molecular structure, which consists of a beta-lactam ring coupled to a monocyclic nucleus. Since they are only effective against a small subset of gram-negative bacteria, these antibiotics are normally reserved for patients who have an allergy to other beta-lactams.

Carbapenem antibiotics are among the few antibiotic classes that can kill both gram-positive and gram-negative bacteria. When other antibiotics have failed to treat an infection, they are often the last resort. Because they include a beta-lactam ring and are resistant to the bacterial enzymes that breakdown this ring, carbapenems are antibiotics that are effective against a wide variety of bacteria.

Beta-lactam antibiotics have the potential to induce serious side effects in some patients, such as allergic responses, gastrointestinal problems, and even liver and kidney damage. A rash is a frequently encountered manifestation of an allergic response, although it is important to note that more severe reactions, such as anaphylaxis, have the potential to result in fatality. Patients with a history of allergy to beta-lactam antibiotics should have close observation for symptoms of an allergic reaction while taking these drugs.

The beta-lactam antibiotics are an effective class of drugs that kill bacteria by stopping them from making their own cell walls. This class of antibiotics includes drugs like penicillin, cephalosporins, monobactams, and carbapenems. The spectrum of activity and resistance to bacterial enzymes possessed by each of these medication types is different. Patients with a known hypersensitivity to beta-lactam antibiotics should have their condition closely checked at all times. These antibiotics have the potential to cause side effects, while being typically safe and effective.

Antibiotics that act on the cell wall

Antibiotics are designed to kill bacteria by attacking their cell wall, which is necessary for the bacterium to survive. Penicillins, cephalosporins, carbapenems, and monobactams are all examples of beta-lactams, a class of antibiotics that specifically targets the cell wall. These antibiotics kill bacteria by preventing their cell walls from being made, which results in their lysis.

Penicillins are one of the first and most popular classes of antibiotics still in use today. They work well against gram-positive and gram-negative bacteria, as well as streptococci and staphylococci. Cephalosporins are used as a secondary treatment for infections that do not respond to penicillin because of their comparable structure and activity. Because of their potency against a wide variety of bacteria, carbapenems are often reserved for the treatment of life-threatening illnesses such hospital-acquired pneumonia and septic shock.

Blockers of protein synthesis

Antibiotics are also effective at halting the protein production process. The ribosomes, the cellular structures responsible for translating genetic code into proteins, are the intended targets of these pharmaceuticals. Antibiotics like aminoglycosides, macrolides, and tetracyclines all share a common property of blocking protein synthesis.

Infections of the urinary tract, respiratory system, and soft tissue are commonly treated with aminoglycosides like gentamicin and streptomycin because they are efficient against gram-negative bacteria. Antibiotics belonging to the macrolide class are efficient against both gram-positive and gram-negative bacteria, making them a popular choice. In addition to treating skin and soft tissue infections, they are frequently used to treat respiratory infections like pneumonia and bronchitis. Similar to penicillin, tetracyclines like doxycycline and minocycline are broad-spectrum antibiotics used to treat a wide variety of bacterial illnesses.

Antifolate drugs

In order for bacteria to thrive and multiply, folic acid metabolism must occur. Sulfonamides and trimethoprim, two antibiotics that interfere with folate metabolism, are efficient against a wide variety of bacteria, both gram-positive and gram-negative. Folic acid is required for DNA replication and cell division, and these medications function by blocking its synthesis.

In the treatment of urinary tract infections, lung infections, and skin and soft tissue infections, sulfonamides like sulfamethoxazole are frequently used in combination with trimethoprim. In addition to treating lung infections, UTIs, and traveler's diarrhea, trimethoprim is often prescribed in combination with sulfamethoxazole.

Anti-mycobacteria drugs

Diseases like tuberculosis and leprosy are caused by mycobacteria. Antibiotics and anti-tuberculosis medications are among those used to treat these conditions. The main purpose of anti-mycobacterial treatment is to eradicate the bacteria and stop the disease from spreading. These medicines are effective because they prevent essential bacterial activities including DNA synthesis, cell wall construction, and protein synthesis from occurring.

Isoniazid is widely used as an anti-mycobacterial medication. Mycolic acids are critical building blocks of the bacterial cell wall, and this medication works by blocking their production. The germs die off and the transmission of tuberculosis is slowed as a result. Rifampin, ethambutol, and pyrazinamide are a few more anti-mycobacterial medicines that see regular use.

Antifungals

Skin, nails, and internal organs are all susceptible to fungal diseases. These infections can be treated with a variety of treatments, both topical and oral. To eliminate the fungus and stop its infection from spreading is the main objective of antifungal treatment.

Fluconazole is widely used as an antifungal medication. This medication is effective because it prevents the production of ergosterol, a lipid required by all fungal cells. This causes the fungus's death and hinders its ability to propagate. Other antifungal medications like itraconazole, ketoconazole, and amphotericin B are also widely used.

Antivirals

Diseases such as the common cold, influenza, and hepatitis can all be caused by viral infections. Drugs that prevent virus replication or block viral entrance into host cells are among those used to treat these infections. Antiviral treatment is administered to lessen the impact of an infection, shorten its duration, and stop its spread.

Acyclovir is widely used as an antiviral medication. The medicine prevents the spread of the herpes simplex virus, which is responsible for both cold sores and genital herpes. Ribavirin is an antiviral medication used to treat hepatitis C, and oseltamivir is an antiviral medication used to treat influenza.

Alkylating agents

Alkylating agents are a class of chemotherapeutic medications that impede DNA replication by adding alkyl groups to the molecule. This stops cancer cells from reproducing and proliferating, which ultimately kills them. Leukemia, lymphoma, breast, and ovarian cancers are only few of the many tumors that alkylating drugs are used to treat.

Cyclophosphamide, ifosfamide, and chlorambucil are all alkylating agents. Side effects like nausea, vomiting, and hair loss can occur because the medications harm healthy cells as well. They are commonly used in combination with other medications, but they remain an essential part of cancer treatment.

Antimetabolites

Antimetabolites are a type of chemotherapy medicine that blocks the ability of cancer cells to make their own DNA and RNA. They achieve this by posing as DNA or RNA building components, which the cancer cell subsequently incorporates into its own DNA or RNA during replication. Because of this disruption, the cancer cell is unable to divide and grow.

Methotrexate, 5-fluorouracil (5-FU), and cytarabine are only some of the antimetabolites that can be found in medicine. Cancers of the breast, lung, and pancreas are only few of the many that these medications treat. Antimetabolites, like alkylating agents, can result in stomach upset, throwing up, and balding.

Natural products

Chemotherapy medications made from natural ingredients are another subset of the field. Cancers that have become resistant to standard chemotherapy treatments are commonly treated with these medications. To be effective, natural compounds disrupt essential cellular division processes as microtubule formation and DNA replication.

Paclitaxel, docetaxel, and vinblastine are all examples of natural product chemotherapeutic medicines. Cancers such as breast cancer, ovarian cancer, and lung cancer are all treated with these medications. However, they may result in negative effects like exhaustion, balding, and nerve damage.

Some of these medications have potential use outside just cancer therapy, including the management of autoimmune disorders including rheumatoid arthritis and lupus. Rheumatoid arthritis, for instance, can be treated with the immunosuppressant methotrexate.

Antibiotics

Antibiotics are a group of medications used to treat infections caused by bacteria. They function by either directly eliminating the germs or blocking their growth. Different types of antibiotics are categorized in accordance with their mode of action, chemical make-up, and therapeutic range. Penicillins, cephalosporins, macrolides, tetracyclines, and fluoroquinolones are only a few examples of widely used classes of antibiotics. The effectiveness and adverse effects of antibiotics depend on the specific bacterium causing the ailment.

Antibiotics aren't the only medications in medicine, though; there are many others.

Others

Drugs that do not fit neatly into any other classification system are included here. Drugs like anticoagulants, which stop blood clots from forming, and antiemetics, which stop vomiting and nausea, are used to treat specific disorders. Nonsteroidal anti-inflammatory medications (NSAIDs) and corticosteroids are used to treat more general symptoms like pain, fever, and inflammation.

Hormonal agents

Hormonal agents are a class of medications that interfere with the endocrine system's ability to regulate growth, metabolism, and sexual development. Estrogens, androgens, progestins, and corticosteroids are all examples of hormonal agents. Hormonal disorders, infertility, and even some forms of cancer can all be treated with these medications.

Preparing and administering oral and parenteral medications

drug preparation and administration are crucial aspects of healthcare that guarantee patients receive the intended therapeutic benefit from their drug. An expert level of training and strict adherence to established protocols are essential for success in this process.

Pills, capsules, and liquids all fall under the category of the oral route of medicine delivery. Verifying the patient's identity, double-checking the drug order, and reviewing the medication's indications, dose, and contraindications prior to oral administration is standard practice. Unless otherwise directed by a doctor or pharmacist, individuals taking oral drugs should be instructed to take them with a full glass of water and not to chew or crush them before swallowing.

Injections into a vein, muscle, or subcutaneous space are the common routes of administration for parenteral drugs. Additional training is necessary for the safe handling of needles, syringes, and other equipment used in the preparation and administration of parenteral drugs. In order to prevent infection and other consequences, healthcare providers must adhere to stringent guidelines when administering the medicine. The identification of the patient must be confirmed, the medicine order checked, and the medication's indications, dosage, and contraindications reviewed before any parenteral medication is given. Needle size and gauge must be chosen carefully, with consideration given to the injection's intended route and intended depth.

Vaccine resources

Vaccination is one of the most effective ways to prevent the spread of infectious illnesses, and healthcare workers play a crucial role in encouraging its use. Vaccines prevent future infections by triggering the immune system to create antibodies against the disease-causing organisms. It is the responsibility of healthcare providers to collaborate with patients to determine whether vaccines are necessary for them depending on their age, current health, and risk factors.

Healthcare practitioners can access vaccine information to assist them keep up with the most recent immunization guidelines and recommendations. Vaccination schedules, vaccine safety, and diseases that can be prevented by vaccination are only few of the topics covered in depth by the Centers for Disease Control and Prevention (CDC). The Centers for Disease Control and Prevention (CDC) also provides numerous training modules and webinars for medical professionals interested in expanding their knowledge of vaccines and their role in public health.

Vaccine information is also available from other sources, including the American Academy of Pediatrics (AAP) and the American College of Obstetricians and Gynecologists (ACOG), respectively. Medical professionals can use these materials to help them give their patients the best possible treatment and guidance..

Chapter 4

General

Common themes in this book's fourth chapter include legal and ethical considerations, effective communication, and the various functions of a healthcare team. In order to offer competent and moral care, these are fundamental concepts that all healthcare providers must grasp.

The healthcare industry is plagued with legal and ethical dilemmas. As medical professionals, it is our duty to act ethically at all times and to comply with all applicable laws and rules. In this section, we'll go through HIPAA, the law that was passed to safeguard patients' private medical records. We will also discuss the need of getting patients' permission before doing any kind of medical operation. Provide the best treatment possible for your patients by learning the laws under which you operate.

When it comes to healthcare, communication is key. Communicating well with patients, family members, and other members of the healthcare team is essential for every healthcare professional. Interpersonal abilities, therapeutic and adaptive reactions, and learning styles will all be discussed in this section. The necessity of professional telephone etiquette and practices, as well as the roles of the health care team, will also be covered.

The chapter concludes by highlighting the value of teamwork among healthcare providers and discussing the many responsibilities that make up a health care team. To guarantee that patients get the best treatment possible, health professionals cannot operate in silos. In this section, we'll learn about the contributions of doctors, nurses, and other healthcare workers.

Understanding the legal and ethical challenges in healthcare, the significance of communication, and working together as a team are all covered in this chapter. Providers who are well-versed in these areas are better able to give their patients the kind of care that is both effective and ethical.

Legal and Ethical Issues

The healthcare industry places a premium on the resolution of legal and ethical concerns. To protect themselves and their employers from legal liability, healthcare providers must be knowledgeable with and compliant with a wide range of laws, regulations, and ethical standards. The Health Insurance Portability and Accountability Act (HIPAA), protected health information (PHI), consent, federal and state regulations, contracts, pharmaceutical laws, mandatory reporting/public health statutes, ethical standards, and medical directives are some of the legal and ethical topics covered in this section. For healthcare providers to meet patients' needs while still adhering to professional and legal guidelines, they must have a firm grasp of these concerns.

Health Insurance Portability and Accountability Act (HIPAA)

While encouraging the electronic interchange of healthcare data, the Health Insurance Portability and Accountability Act (HIPAA) of 1996 was enacted to safeguard patients' personal health information (PHI). Patients are guaranteed access to their own medical records and electronic billing and claims processes are standardized thanks to HIPAA.

The Privacy Rule is an essential part of HIPAA since it specifies rules for the handling of protected health information. Healthcare providers and health insurance companies are examples of covered entities that are obligated to take measures to preserve the privacy of patients' protected health information (PHI). Patients should be informed of their rights to access and amend their health records and other privacy protections.

The Security Rule was established by HIPAA to preserve the privacy, accuracy, and availability of electronic protected health information (PHI) held by covered businesses. This includes using encryption and audit measures to prevent unwanted access to electronic PHI.

The Department of Health and Human Services can now investigate and punish HIPAA violators thanks to the Enforcement Rule. Noncompliance can result in serious consequences, including monetary fines and even jail time in the case of criminal breaches.

The breach notification regulations of the Health Insurance Portability and Accountability Act (HIPAA) require covered companies to inform individuals affected by a breach of unsecured protected health information. The Department of Health and Human Services must also be notified when a breach occurs at a covered organization.

Providing national guidelines for the protection of PHI and encouraging the electronic sharing of healthcare data, HIPAA has had a profound effect on the healthcare system. Covered entities now have additional duties, such as notifying affected individuals and enforcing appropriate administrative, physical, and technical precautions to protect personal health information (PHI).

Protected Health Information (PHI)

Information about an individual's health that is created, received, maintained, or transferred by a covered entity or its business associate is considered Protected Health Information (PHI). The HIPAA Privacy Rule lays out strict guidelines for how medical professionals can use and disclose patients' personal health information (PHI) while still protecting their confidentiality.

Individuals' names, addresses, Social Security numbers, medical record numbers, and other identifying numbers and characteristics are all examples of PHI. Physical and mental health records, health care service records, and financial records are all considered protected health information. Information such as medical histories, test findings, treatment plans, medication lists, prescriptions, and bills are examples of PHI.

Health insurance companies, health care providers, and health care clearinghouses are all examples of "covered entities" that are obligated by HIPAA to take measures to protect the privacy, security, and accessibility of their patients' protected health information (PHI). A notice of privacy practices detailing the ways in which protected health information (PHI) may be used and shared, as well as the patient's rights to access and control such information, must be provided to patients by covered entities. In addition, in order to use or disclose a patient's PHI for marketing or research purposes, a covered entity must first receive the patient's written authorization.

In order to prevent any misuse or exposure of protected health information (PHI), HIPAA mandates that all covered entities put in place appropriate administrative, physical, and technical safeguards. Policies and procedures for accessing and utilizing PHI, training for employees, and periodic risk assessments are all examples of administrative protections. Locked doors and cabinets are examples of physical security measures that can be taken to prevent unauthorized access to protected health information. When it comes to protecting sensitive data during transmission over the internet, technical precautions include things like firewalls and encryption.

Violators of HIPAA face harsh consequences, including imprisonment and annual fines of up to $1.5 million. In order to ensure compliance with HIPAA standards, covered entities must take the protection of PHI seriously and develop detailed policies and procedures.

Other laws and regulations, in addition to HIPAA, govern the privacy of patients' medical records. Substance addiction patients are afforded extra privacy safeguards by legislation like the Confidentiality of Alcohol and Drug addiction Patient Records (42 CFR Part 2). The Genetic Information Nondiscrimination Act (GINA) prohibits health insurers and prospective employers from making determinations or judgments based on an individual's genetic composition.

The privacy and confidentiality of patients' health records depend on the safeguarding of PHI. In addition to installing safeguards to protect PHI against unauthorized access, use, or disclosure, covered entities must take proactive actions to assure compliance with HIPAA and other applicable laws and regulations. Furthermore, it is imperative to provide patients with comprehensive guidelines elucidating the manner in which their personal health information will be utilized and divulged.

Consent

The idea of autonomy, which acknowledges that patients have the right to make decisions about their health and well-being, is the basis for consent, a basic part of medical practice. In order to obtain a patient's "informed consent," doctors must explain their diagnosis, the planned treatment, and any risks or advantages to the patient. Before administering care or performing operations, medical professionals must have the patient's permission to do so.

Medical professionals have a moral and legal duty to protect the rights of their patients by obtaining informed consent before performing any procedure. Patients' vocal, written, or even nonverbal actions might be used to get consent. Consent is not merely a form to be signed; rather, it is a process of continuous dialogue between the healthcare professional and the patient.

Valid permission requires the three pillars of being freely provided by an informed, capable individual. The term "voluntary consent" refers to an agreement that was reached without any pressure or improper influence. The patient must be given an accurate and comprehensive explanation of their medical condition, the planned therapy, and the risks and advantages of the treatment in order to give their informed consent. In order for the patient to make an educated choice regarding their care, the healthcare provider must give them all of the relevant information. The patient has the mental and legal capacity to provide their permission.

In cases of emergency where the patient is unable to give consent or where the treatment is mandated by law, consent is not required and may be waived. Still, healthcare providers have an ethical obligation to prioritize the patient's best interests wherever possible.

In healthcare contexts, it is possible to gain many forms of permission. The term "express consent" refers to when a patient gives their full and unqualified approval for a medical procedure. A patient's actions or the nature of their medical condition can be used to infer their implied consent. A patient's action of extending an arm for a nurse to draw blood, for instance, could be construed as implicit permission for the blood draw.

When dealing with vulnerable populations like minors, people with cognitive disabilities, or patients who do not speak the language of the healthcare professional, gaining consent can be very difficult. Healthcare practitioners should take special precautions to ensure that patients in these situations completely comprehend the proposed treatment and its related risks and benefits.

In addition to being required by law, obtaining consent is also the ethical thing to do for medical professionals. Providers of medical treatment have a responsibility to foster an atmosphere conducive to patient participation in decision-making regarding their care. This involves doing things like giving patients information in a way that they can understand, communicating honestly and openly with them, and giving them space to make their own decisions.

Medical professionals have a moral and legal responsibility to ensure their patients are fully informed before they consent to treatment. It necessitates that patients be given the opportunity to make an informed decision about their healthcare and that they be given sufficient information about their medical condition and treatment alternatives. The permission procedure must be voluntary and granted by a competent individual, and healthcare practitioners must ensure these conditions.

Federal and state regulations

The healthcare industry relies heavily on federal and state laws. They are put in place to guarantee that healthcare providers and institutions are adhering to appropriate norms of practice and protecting the public's health from harm. The federal government creates federal regulations, whereas states create their own regulations. Both types of rules are necessary to protect patients' health and well-being.

Federal Regulations

The healthcare industry is heavily regulated by the federal government. Federal healthcare regulations are enforced by multiple departments and agencies, including the Centers for Medicare & Medicaid Services (CMS), the Food and Drug Administration (FDA), and the Department of Health and Human Services (HHS).

The Centers for Medicare & Medicaid Services (CMS) manages and enforces federal healthcare laws and policies, such as Medicare and Medicaid. The agency is responsible for ensuring that healthcare facilities meet quality standards and for certifying and accrediting those facilities.

Drugs, medical devices, and other types of healthcare products are subject to oversight by the Food and Drug Administration (FDA). The organization checks the quality and safety of products on the market to ensure they are fit for consumers.

The Department of Health and Human Services (HHS) is in charge of enforcing HIPAA and other healthcare privacy and security laws. The CDC, whose job it is to keep an eye on public health and stop the spread of disease, is under the agency's purview as well.

State Regulations

Each state also has its own healthcare laws in addition to those at the federal level. Patients' health and safety are essential concerns for states, thus they regulate the healthcare industry to make sure doctors and institutions follow the law.

Standards for healthcare delivery, as well as the certification and licensing of healthcare providers and facilities, may be mandated by individual states. For instance, in order to keep their licenses current, medical professionals in some states must complete an annual minimum number of hours of continuing education. Some states may mandate periodic inspections of healthcare facilities to verify their conformance with mandates.

Contracts

Relationships, both professional and personal, rely heavily on contracts. Contracts are crucial in the healthcare industry because they guarantee the provision of adequate services and safeguard the interests of all parties. A contract is a formal, written agreement between at least two parties that sets down the responsibilities and rights of each of them. While verbal agreements are acceptable, written contracts are preferred since they serve as a permanent record of the agreement and lessen the likelihood of misunderstandings or legal problems arising out of the terms of the contract.

Providers, patients, insurers, and suppliers are just some of the possible participants in a healthcare contract. Employer agreements, service contracts, rental agreements for medical tools, and managed care contracts are all commonplace in the healthcare industry. When engaging into any contract, healthcare providers must adhere to all applicable federal and state rules.

Healthcare providers and their staff members enter into employment contracts. The employment obligations, pay, benefits, and termination provisions are all spelled out in the contract. Employment contracts should include terms addressing discrimination, harassment, and other concerns connected to employment in accordance with federal and state labor regulations.

Cleaning services, medical transcription, and information technology assistance are all examples of services for which healthcare providers and vendors enter into contracts. Contracts for services should detail not just what will be provided, but also the terms under which those services will be provided, paid for, and even ended. HIPAA and OSHA are two examples of standards that healthcare providers should check their vendors' compliance with before signing a contract with them.

Medical imaging and diagnostic tools, as well as patient monitoring devices, are only few examples of the types of equipment for which providers and suppliers enter into rental agreements. The rental terms and conditions, including the rental period, rental rates, maintenance tasks, and liability for damages, should all be included in the contract. If a healthcare professional purchases medical equipment, they should double check that it conforms with all applicable standards, such as those imposed by the Food and Drug Administration.

Healthcare providers and managed care organizations or insurance companies enter into managed care contracts to coordinate patient care. Covered services, payment rates, and quality indicators are all factors that are specified in these contracts for the delivery of healthcare. Providers of medical services should examine such agreements thoroughly to guarantee compliance with applicable laws and safeguarding of their financial interests.

Healthcare providers have a responsibility beyond just meeting legal requirements to ensure that any contracts they enter into are moral and consistent with their core beliefs. Contract ethics involve things like making sure patients get the care they need, keeping their information private, avoiding conflicts of interest, and getting their approval before doing anything. In addition, healthcare providers should check that their contracts are easy to understand and follow.

Healthcare providers should consult with attorneys and other professionals to verify that their contracts are both legal and ethical. Healthcare attorneys are useful resources for questions about federal and state rules, as well as for drafting and reviewing contracts. The American Medical Association and the American Nurses Association are two organizations that can give healthcare providers with advice on ethical matters related to contracts.

Quality healthcare cannot be provided without contracts, which also serve to safeguard the interests of all parties. Providers of medical services have a moral and legal obligation to do business in accordance with applicable state and federal laws. Healthcare providers that seek professional and legal counsel are better able to write and review contracts in accordance with the law and professional standards.

Medical regulation

Pharmaceutical laws are the set of rules that control how medicine is made, sold, and used. The public's health and the integrity of the pharmaceutical industry depend on these regulations. In the United States, the Food and Drug Administration (FDA) is responsible for enforcing pharmaceutical rules, while in Europe it is the European Medicines Agency (EMA) and in many other countries it is the Ministry of Health.

Making sure drugs are safe and effective for patients is a major focus of pharmaceutical legislation. Pharmaceutical laws do this by dictating minimum requirements for the safety testing, production, labeling, and packaging of pharmaceuticals. Drugs that are free of contamination, satisfy adequate potency and purity requirements, and have accurate packaging and labeling thanks to these regulations. These regulations also mandate comprehensive testing and examination of all pharmaceuticals by regulatory agencies prior to their approval for use in patients.

The distribution and advertising of pharmaceuticals are likewise governed by legislation. It is against the law in many countries for pharmaceutical firms to advertise their products for applications not approved by the FDA. Companies cannot make any claims about the safety or effectiveness of their products that cannot be proven under these laws. Additionally, pharmaceutical regulations lay forth guidelines for drug price and reimbursement, and some of these drugs may be mandated to be provided to patients at reduced or no cost.

Pharmacist and pharmacy oversight is another critical component of pharmaceutical legislation. Requirements for licensure, credentials of staff, and record-keeping are all established by these statutes. In addition, they lay forth guidelines for the distribution of medications, such as what must be done in terms of drug labeling, patient education, and the custody of controlled substances.

Pharmaceutical laws not only govern the manufacturing and distribution of pharmaceuticals, but also the usage of medical devices like diagnostic tests, imaging machines, and other tools utilized in the medical field. These regulations help guarantee that all manufactured and distributed medical devices are up to par with patient safety and efficacy requirements.

The Food and Drug Administration (FDA) of the United States is one example of a government agency tasked with enforcing pharmaceutical rules. These departments have the authority to conduct inspections of pharmaceutical facilities, conduct investigations of consumer complaints, and take legal action against businesses and persons that break the law. The consequences of breaking these rules range from monetary fines and license suspensions to criminal prosecution.

Pharmaceutical law is dynamic, changing to accommodate new scientific discoveries, medical procedures, and public health concerns. Complex medications generated from living creatures, such as biologics, have received more attention from regulators in recent years. It is crucial that pharmaceutical regulations continue to improve to ensure that patients receive safe, effective, and reasonably priced care as the pharmaceutical sector innovates and develops new products and treatments.

Mandatory reporting/public health statutes

Healthcare practitioners and other professionals are required by law to report certain disorders or diseases to public health authorities in accordance with mandatory reporting and public health statutes. In order to safeguard public health and stop the spread of contagious diseases, certain laws have been enacted. They also aid in the monitoring and tracking of outbreaks by health authorities and in the preparation of public health emergencies.

However, some disorders are reported to the federal government regardless of state laws governing mandatory reporting and public health. While the CDC has issued recommendations on how to handle public health emergencies, it is ultimately the duty of state and local governments.

Infectious diseases like tuberculosis, hepatitis, STDs, and food poisoning are frequently reported under obligatory reporting and public health regulations. Child abuse, neglect, domestic violence, and work-related illnesses and injuries may also warrant reporting.

Certain conditions must be reported by healthcare providers and other professionals upon diagnosis or suspicion. Cases of bioterrorism or other public health emergencies must also be reported. If these issues aren't reported, you could face fines and other legal repercussions.

Both the conditions that must be reported and the procedure for doing so differ from state to state. Cases of reportable conditions must be reported by healthcare practitioners to the appropriate state or local public health agency. This can be done via telephone, fax, or an electronic reporting system. Additional patient data, including providers' names, ages, and contact details, may be requested.

When a report is made, public health officials have the option of conducting an investigation to stop the disease from spreading further. Public health interventions may involve isolating or quarantining the patient and any contacts they may have, as well as educating the patient and their contacts.

Challenges and restrictions might be found in required reporting and public health laws. Underreporting or late reporting of cases is a problem that could hinder public health efforts to contain epidemics. Because some medical problems are stigmatized or lead to prejudice, there is also a risk of confidentiality breaches.

Protecting the public health and avoiding the spread of infectious diseases requires the use of instruments such as mandatory reporting and public health regulations. Cases of reportable conditions must be reported by healthcare practitioners and other professionals to the appropriate state or local public health agency. Authorities in the field of public health can better protect the health of their communities and identify and contain outbreaks if they work together.

Ethical standards

Professionals and laypeople alike can look to ethical standards as a set of guiding principles for making morally and socially sound choices. For healthcare to be effective, safe, and respectful of patients' rights and dignity, ethical norms must be adhered to at all times. Providers of healthcare services benefit greatly from having a framework for dealing with ethical dilemmas and conflicts of interest that may occur in the course of their job. Some of the most important ethical norms in healthcare will be discussed below.

Autonomy

The term "autonomy" is used to describe an individual's right to determine his or her own medical treatment. Some examples of these rights are the ability to provide or withhold permission to medical treatment and have a voice in how those decisions are made. As part of their duty to their patients, healthcare professionals must give them all the facts they need to make educated decisions about their treatment.

Beneficence

Medical professionals have a duty of beneficence to prioritize their patients' health and well-being above all else. Treatments must be successful, harm must be avoided, and health must be promoted. Providers of healthcare must strike a balance between doing no harm to their patients and acting in a beneficent manner.

Non-maleficence

To practice non-maleficence means to have a duty to cause no harm to one's patients. This involves declining potentially harmful treatments or interventions that are not in the patient's best interests. Providers of healthcare must strike a balance between non-maleficence and beneficence, or the duty to improve patients' lives.

Justice

When we talk about justice in healthcare, we're talking about the duty of doctors and nurses to treat all patients fairly and equally, regardless of their background or beliefs. This involves making sure that everyone, regardless of financial means, has access to the medical attention they need.

Fidelity

The term "fidelity" is used to describe the duty of healthcare workers to remain loyal and trustworthy to their patients. Keeping patients' information private, treating them with dignity, and adhering to all applicable regulations are all part of this.

Veracity

The duty of healthcare providers to tell their patients the truth is known as veracity. Included in this is the disclosure of any potential biases or conflicts of interest that may affect their care, as well as the provision of accurate information about diagnosis, therapies, and prognoses.

Informed consent

Patients are better able to make decisions about their health when they have all the facts regarding their diagnosis, potential treatments, risks, and benefits. After then, it is the patient's prerogative to make an educated choice about their treatment. Consent with full knowledge and understanding is a cornerstone of ethical behavior and a legal requirement in many countries.

Confidentiality

Providers in the medical field have a duty of confidentiality to their patients to prevent the misuse of their private information. Except when disclosure is compelled by law or essential to protect the patient or others from harm, healthcare providers are obligated to maintain strict confidentiality.

End-of-life care

When a patient is terminally ill or nearing the end of their existence, they need special care known as end-of-life care. Treatment with life-sustaining measures, their removal, and the provision of palliative care to alleviate pain and other symptoms all fall under the umbrella of end-of-life care ethics.

Healthcare professionals must always operate ethically. In order to ensure that their patients receive treatment that meets these standards, healthcare professionals must be familiar with them and work to implement them into daily practice. Those in the medical field can do more for the people they treat and the communities they live in by adhering to ethical principles.

Medical directives

In order to help doctors decide how to manage their patients, medical directives are often used. When a patient is unable to communicate their wishes to their healthcare providers, a medical directive can be used to outline their preferences for treatment in advance. They are also commonly referred to as "living wills" or "advance directives."

When a patient is unable to express their preferences for medical care, a medical directive can be used to honor those wishes regardless of the patient's condition. Written documents, videos, audio recordings, and spoken directions given to an authorized representative (often a family member or close friend) are all valid types of medical directives.

End-of-life care wishes, such as whether or not the patient wants to receive life-sustaining therapies like mechanical breathing or cardiopulmonary resuscitation (CPR), are commonly included in medical directives. Instructions for dealing with suffering, organ donation, and funeral preparations are also possible.

Many people make their advance directives for healthcare long before they ever need them. As long as the patient retains legal decision-making capacity, they can control their own medical treatment. Patients and their loved ones can rest easy knowing their desires will be followed.

Directives for medical treatment are legally binding and recognized in all but a handful of states. However, medical directive laws are not uniform across the country. Some jurisdictions require notarization or witnessing of signatures. In other countries, just giving someone verbal instructions is enough.

As long as they don't violate professional standards of care or the law, healthcare providers must honor patients' advance directives. A healthcare professional may face legal consequences if they disobey a patient's advance directives.

Healthcare providers should be familiar with the legal and ethical considerations of medical directives because of the complexity and sensitivity of the subject matter. They need to be able to help patients and their loved ones understand healthcare directives so that they may make well-informed decisions.

Patients can make decisions about their care while they are still competent, and their wishes can be honored even if they lose that capacity thanks to medical directives. Providers of medical care have a professional and legal obligation to comply with patients' advance directives.

Communication

Delivering top-notch healthcare relies heavily on clear and constant communication between all involved parties. In order to give the greatest care possible, the medical staff must be able to talk to each other and their patients. The success of treatment plans, the level of patient happiness, and the efficacy of healthcare delivery are all affected by the communicative abilities of healthcare professionals.

Interpersonal and therapeutic/adaptive reactions, learning styles, healthcare team roles, and professional telephone etiquette/techniques will all be discussed in this part as they pertain to the field of healthcare communication.

Interpersonal relationship skills

Communication and teamwork in the healthcare industry rely heavily on employees' interpersonal abilities. Having strong interpersonal skills is essential for delivering excellent care and achieving the best possible health outcomes with patients and their loved ones. In this section, we'll talk about why it's crucial for healthcare professionals to have strong interpersonal skills, what such skills consist of, and how to hone them.

Importance of Interpersonal Relationship Skills in Healthcare

In order to offer good care, connect with patients and their families, and earn their trust, healthcare workers need strong interpersonal relationship skills. Effective communication skills are essential for fostering supportive connections with patients and coworkers in the healthcare setting, which may be high-pressure and emotionally fraught. Positive patient outcomes, higher levels of patient satisfaction, and fewer medical mistakes have all been linked to healthcare professionals with strong interpersonal skills.

Key Components of Interpersonal Relationship Skills

There are several facets to effective interpersonal relationship skills.

Active listening

The ability to listen attentively and respond appropriately is crucial in every kind of conversation. Active listening entails focusing on what the other person is saying, asking questions to get more information, and giving suggestions for improvement. Trust, mutual regard, and efficient problem-solving are all aided by attentive listening.

Empathy

To have empathy is to feel and comprehend what other people are going through. When medical staff show compassion for their patients and their loved ones, it strengthens the bonds between them and ultimately improves the quality of treatment provided. Medical personnel that are able to empathize with their patients are better able to treat them.

Effective communication

Interpersonal ties in healthcare are only as strong as their ability to communicate effectively. Trust, fewer misunderstandings, and better patient outcomes are all the results of communication that is clear, succinct, and courteous. Listening attentively, having compassion, and articulating complex concepts in layman's terms are all necessary components of effective communication with patients and their loved ones.

Conflict resolution

The ability to handle and resolve disagreement in a courteous and constructive manner is an essential part of having strong interpersonal interaction skills, which are frequent in the healthcare industry. To resolve a conflict in the healthcare setting, experts need to be able to pinpoint its origin, show respect for opposing viewpoints, and work together to find a solution that everyone can live with.

Strategies for Developing Interpersonal Relationship Skills

There are a number of methods that may be used to better a person's interpersonal relationship abilities, which are crucial for healthcare practitioners.

Self-awareness

To be self-aware, one must comprehend their own feelings, prejudices, and method of expression. Improving one's interpersonal skills is as simple as becoming more self-aware, taking stock of one's own strengths and limitations, and actively seeking feedback from one's peers and patients.

Active listening practice

Active listening is a skill that can help healthcare personnel connect with patients and each other. Healthcare providers can improve their communication abilities and earn the respect of their peers by listening attentively to their patients and coworkers.

Role-playing

When done in a safe setting, role-playing can be a useful tool for honing one's social skills. To better their communication and conflict resolution abilities, healthcare professionals might practice scenarios with coworkers or in training sessions.

Professional development

Workshops, conferences, and other forms of professional development training can aid healthcare professionals in honing their interpersonal skills. These occasions offer the chance to acquire the knowledge and practice of interpersonal skills such as effective communication and conflict resolution.

Relational competence is crucial for those working in healthcare because it facilitates open lines of communication, fosters patient trust, and encourages compassionate treatment. improved patient care, fewer errors in the operating room, and improved long-term health outcomes are all possible when healthcare personnel acquire these abilities. The interpersonal skills of healthcare professionals can be enhanced through self-awareness training, active listening exercises, role-playing, and participation in professional development opportunities.

Therapeutic/adaptive responses

Therapeutic and adaptive reactions are the tools and strategies used by medical practitioners to meet their patients' emotional, cognitive, and behavioral requirements. The objective of these comments is to make the hospital experience more positive and empowering for the patients so that they may better manage their health.

Therapeutic and adaptive responses necessitate sensitivity, attentiveness, and fluency in speech. The capacity to connect with patients is crucial for successful treatment. The ability to empathize with patients and fully grasp their circumstances is essential for every healthcare worker.

Active listening is a powerful therapeutic and adaptive response. Paying attentive attention to the patient, asking them questions to help you better understand what they're saying, and giving them positive comments are all examples of active listening. Using this method, therapists and patients are more likely to develop the trusting, collaborative relationships necessary for effective treatment.

Validation is another powerful method. Validation is the process of validating the patient's feelings and emotions and communicating that they are appropriate and valid. The healthcare professional can aid in the patient's recovery by validating the patient's emotions. When the patient is experiencing strong feelings like anxiety or terror, validation can be especially beneficial.

Cognitive and behavioral approaches are another tool available to healthcare providers for assisting patients in managing their diseases. One such method is cognitive-behavioral therapy (CBT), which targets both the patient's ideas and actions. Depression, anxiety, and substance misuse are just some of the many disorders that can be helped by cognitive behavioral therapy. Healthcare providers can improve patients' health outcomes by assisting them in recognizing and altering unproductive patterns of thought and action.

Other therapeutic and adaptive responses include problem-solving and goal-setting sessions, as well as motivational interviewing. Patients who have doubts about modifying their behavior can benefit from a practice called motivational interviewing. In cases where patients may be reluctant to change, including when trying to quit smoking or cut back on alcohol intake, this method is frequently employed. Patients can be assisted in determining what is preventing them from reaching their health objectives and in creating a strategy for doing so through the use of problem-solving and goal-setting strategies.

Understanding the patient's requirements, motives, and preferences is crucial for providing effective treatment and adaptive responses. Medical professionals should be able to evaluate a patient's health, address their concerns, and offer guidance and advice. Successful outcomes are highly dependent on the therapist's ability to form a good rapport with the patient.

It's important to remember that the therapeutic and coping processes at play in healthcare settings extend beyond the patient-provider dynamic. These abilities are transferable to other areas of healthcare, such as team-based treatment. The ability of healthcare teams to effectively communicate, work together, and solve problems is crucial to the delivery of high-quality treatment.

Healthcare relies heavily on therapeutic and adaptive responses. It takes a multifaceted set of abilities for healthcare professionals to meet the emotional, psychological, and physiological demands of their patients. Healthcare practitioners need to have abilities including active listening, validating patients' experiences, and using cognitive and behavioral strategies. Providers can improve their patients' health outcomes and quality of life by making use of these abilities.

Learning styles

Each person has a unique "learning style" that affects how they absorb and use information. One's own learning style influences how effectively one takes in and remembers new information. Educators and trainers can improve student results by developing a deeper understanding of how different learners process information. In this article, we'll examine the many pedagogical approaches known as "learning styles" and how they can facilitate better education.

In terms of how people learn, visual, auditory, and kinesthetic are the most frequent preferences. Those who are "visual learners" like to take in information via visual means, such as photos, diagrams, films, etc. They are more likely to remember data given graphically. However, those who are "auditory learners" prefer to take in information by auditory means. They learn best through auditory means such as lectures, group discussions, and podcasts. Those who learn best through movement and physical interaction are called kinesthetic learners. Information learned through simulations, role-playing, and other interactive activities is more easily retained by this group.

There are more, less well-known, but no less significant learning styles than the aforementioned three. Some students, for instance, are what we call "verbal learners," who acquire knowledge best through conversation and writing. Some students, called social learners, do better in a classroom setting or with other people around. Finally, there are students that thrive in an ad hoc, self-directed learning environment.

However, some people may have a dominant learning style that shapes their preferences, and most people have a mix of learning styles. A pupil might, for instance, be more of a visual learner than an auditory or tactile one. Educators and trainers can better meet the demands of their students if they have a firm grasp of the many learning styles at their disposal.

To better communicate with their patients, healthcare professionals should be aware of and accommodate for a variety of patient learning styles. Healthcare practitioners should adapt their communication strategies to each patient's individual preferences and learning styles. A patient who learns best visually, for instance, would benefit from diagrams, drawings, or films, whereas a patient who learns best aurally might favor talks or lectures.

In addition, healthcare personnel can benefit greatly from furthering their own education and development by increasing their awareness of and facility with various learning styles. In order to deliver the highest quality treatment for their patients, healthcare professionals must continually expand their expertise. If medical professionals take the time to identify their preferred method of learning, they will be better able to select the most effective methods of continuing their education.

Educators, trainers, and healthcare practitioners would all benefit from a deeper understanding of the variety of learning styles that exists among their patients and clients. Healthcare providers can better communicate with patients and further their own professional growth if they are aware of and able to accommodate a variety of learning styles.

Health care team roles

Quality patient care requires the collaborative efforts of many in today's healthcare system. These people, collectively known as the healthcare team, play crucial roles in ensuring positive patient outcomes. The many members of the healthcare team and their respective contributions to patient care will be discussed below.

Physician

The doctor is a qualified medical expert who can make diagnoses and provide treatments. They might work at a clinic or hospital and have a focus like pediatrics or cardiology.

Nurse

The nurse is a qualified medical expert who assists doctors in caring for patients. Nurses play a crucial role in healthcare by keeping tabs on patients, doling out medication, and comforting both patients and their loved ones. They might also aid in the creation of care plans and patient education materials.

Pharmacist

The pharmacist's duties include delivering medication and educating patients and other medical professionals on its proper use. They may also collaborate with doctors to create treatment programs that incorporate medication and track patients' progress.

Physical Therapist

A physical therapist is a medical doctor who specializes in diagnosing and treating people who are having trouble moving around. They may help those who have been hurt or who have just undergone surgery get back on their feet.

Occupational Therapist

Restoring functional independence in patients with physical, mental, and cognitive impairments is a primary goal for the occupational therapist. Patients who have had a stroke or been given a chronic illness diagnosis may be among those they work with.

Speech-Language Pathologist

A speech-language pathologist is a medical doctor who specializes in diagnosing and treating people who have trouble communicating. They may interact with those who have trouble communicating because of illness or injury.

Medical Assistant

A medical assistant is a type of healthcare worker who assists doctors and other medical professionals in a variety of settings. They might collect vital signs, give out medications, and aid in other administrative tasks.

Patient Care Technician

Patient care technicians are members of the medical staff who assist nurses in their duties. They can provide basic medical care and aid with activities of daily living including bathing and clothing.

Social Worker

The social worker's job is to assist patients and their loved ones in understanding and making the most of their options within the hospital system. Patients and their families suffering with a chronic disease or disability may also be offered counseling and support services.

Each of these positions on the healthcare team is crucial to the successful treatment of patients. The finest treatment for patients and better outcomes can be achieved when medical professionals collaborate and share their knowledge and experience.

Professional telephone etiquette/techniques

The telephone is widely used as a key means of communication in healthcare settings, highlighting the importance of clear and concise speech. Proper telephone etiquette is essential for effective two-way communication between medical staff and patients, as well as within healthcare teams. Effective and efficient telephone communication can go a long way toward preventing miscommunication, blunders, and problems in the workplace.

Answering the Phone

One of the cornerstones of polite phone behavior is a prompt response when the phone rings. The standard response time for answering a phone is three rings, or 15 seconds. The individual who answers the phone for the medical facility should introduce themselves and state their position. You might hear something like, "Good morning, this is Nurse Smith on the sixth floor." Not only does this let the caller know who they're talking to, but it also confirms that they've dialed the right number.

Active Listening

When having a conversation over the phone, it is crucial to listen attentively. Active listening entails paying close attention to the speaker, taking in what they are saying, and then checking to see if you both understand each other. By listening attentively, you can avoid miscommunication and better serve the caller.

Avoid Distractions

When answering the phone, focus on the person on the other end and do your best to block out any background noise. This includes muting the TV or radio and minimizing unnecessary distractions like other people talking. The caller should be the only thing on the mind of the person answering the phone.

Tone of Voice

Good telephone manners include being aware of and adjusting one's tone of voice accordingly. An anxious and irritated patient is no match for a doctor who speaks in a soothing, comforting tone. Building rapport and trust with a caller requires an approachable, helpful, and professional tone.

Confidentiality

Telephone interactions must be treated as confidential in the healthcare industry. Only the patient or a member of the patient's immediate family should be given confidential health information over the phone. Before giving out any personal information, it's smart to be sure you can trust the person on the other end of the line.

Taking Messages

It's vital that you take careful notes when taking a phone message. Everything from the caller's name and number to the patient's details and the message itself must be recorded, as well as any necessary follow-up. Reiterating the message back to the caller for verification is also crucial.

Ending the Call

Just as crucial as answering the phone is ending it in a professional manner. The last person on the call should provide a brief summary of the discussion and confirm any next steps that were discussed. The caller should be thanked for contacting the healthcare team and offered assistance moving forward.

Proper use of the telephone is crucial for efficient communication in the medical field. Building rapport and trust over the phone can help cut down on miscommunication and increase productivity. By adhering to these standards, medical staff will be able to better communicate with one another and give superior care to their patients.

Chapter 5

Administrative

A dministrative duties are essential to the efficient running of any healthcare organization. Billing and coding, appointment scheduling, and data accuracy are just a few of the many tasks that fall on the shoulders of healthcare executives and personnel. These administrative duties guarantee that patients will receive the safest and most effective care available.

This section serves as an introduction to the fundamental responsibilities of healthcare administrators. We'll go over billing and coding procedures, insurance plans, patient service coverage, fee reductions, and exemptions. We will also discuss financial terms, billing/collections processes, and patient account financial procedures.

Appointment scheduling and data accuracy are as important as billing and coding in the healthcare industry. The way doctors and hospitals keep track of patient data has been completely transformed with the advent of electronic health records (EHRs). We'll talk about electronic health records (EHRs) and other electronic charting and file systems that can help medical facilities better manage patient records.

In-depth knowledge of the essential administrative activities necessary for the smooth operation of a healthcare facility is provided in this chapter. It will aid medical personnel in providing the highest quality care to patients while meeting all legal and financial obligations.

Billing, Coding and Insurance

Healthcare would not function without billing, coding, and insurance. Accurate coding and billing are essential to the financial well-being of both healthcare professionals and their patients. Healthcare practitioners face the additional challenge of keeping up with ever-changing billing and insurance policies and procedures. In this chapter, you'll get an overview of such topics as financial terms, patient account financial procedures, billing, and collections; insurance coding and fraud; insurance coverage for patient services; and more. Professionals in the healthcare field can better serve their patients and comply with applicable requirements if they have a firm grasp of the ins and outs of billing, coding, and insurance.

Coding applications

Healthcare billing and reimbursement rely heavily on coding application software. Coding is used in healthcare to keep track of patients' procedures, diagnoses, and treatments. The two most used coding systems in healthcare are the ICD and CPT, and it is from these that billing and payment codes are derived. Healthcare professionals can get paid what they're worth thanks to these coding systems, which facilitate precise patient-service billing and payment.

CPT codes are used to describe the medical services and treatments that were rendered, while ICD codes are used to identify and report medical diagnoses. Accurate billing and reimbursement are made possible by the widespread adoption of these codes, which standardize the reporting of medical diagnoses and operations. Providers may do more with patient data and outcomes, illness prevalence tracking, and clinical decision making when using standardized codes.

Those working in healthcare must be well-versed in the coding systems in use at their facilities, as well as the standards and regulations that govern the coding process. Accurate documentation in support of allocated codes is essential, and this requires familiarity with the requirements for coding specificity. Correct coding and billing can only be achieved via proper training and ongoing education.

Coding and billing have been made much simpler thanks to EHR technology. By eliminating the need for paper records and increasing efficiency, electronic health records (EHRs) have revolutionized the healthcare industry. Electronic health records (EHRs) also help doctors keep tabs on their patients' outcomes and conduct in-depth analyses of their data.

Despite their importance in healthcare billing and reimbursement, coding programs can be exploited for fraudulent purposes. Both patients and healthcare providers risk losing money due to improper payments or overpayments caused by billing and coding mistakes, whether those mistakes are deliberate or not. Therefore, it is crucial that medical staff understand the regulations and policies governing billing and coding, as well as the potential repercussions of engaging in fraudulent practices.

Accurate medical billing and reimbursement depend on the use of coding software. They aid in the precise recording of medical procedures, as well as the reporting and subsequent analysis of patient data and their outcomes. But healthcare providers also need to be alert to the possibility of fraud and abuse and make sure they adhere to norms and regulations when assigning codes.

Insurance fraud and/or abuse

There are a wide variety of methods that can be used to commit insurance fraud or abuse in the healthcare sector. Abuse refers to behaviors that are not in accordance with generally accepted standards of medical, business, or financial conduct, whereas fraud refers to the intentional misrepresenting of facts for financial advantage. Legal, financial, and moral repercussions can all result from healthcare fraud and abuse.

Insurance billing fraud is a widespread problem in the healthcare industry. This might happen if doctors or hospitals try to get paid for services that weren't actually performed on the patient or weren't covered by their insurance. Providers that "upcode," or overstate the seriousness of a patient's ailment, in order to earn greater payment rates, are also guilty of billing fraud.

Insurance fraud also occurs in the realm of pharmaceuticals. This may occur if doctors overprescribe or prescribe medications that aren't necessary just to earn a profit from the pharmaceutical industry.

However, there are numerous types of insurance fraud. In order to boost their bottom lines, some doctors prescribe more tests and procedures than are really necessary. Patients and health insurance providers may end up spending more than necessary as a result of this. The term "unbundling" refers to the practice of providers charging customers for each component of a service separately rather than for the entire package.

Healthcare providers and institutions should implement and strictly adhere to policies and procedures designed to avoid insurance fraud and abuse. It is the responsibility of the providers to guarantee that they are correctly billing for their services and that they are only prescribing treatments and medications that are actually needed. Insurance billing and prescription procedures have specific legal requirements that providers must meet.

Fraud and abuse prevention is a priority for insurance firms as well. By doing checks like audits and reviews of billing procedures, they can uncover and prevent fraudulent actions. They can inform consumers about their insurance benefits and the significance of reporting suspicious activity, and they can collaborate with healthcare providers to establish best practices for prescription and invoicing.

The repercussions of insurance fraud and misuse in the healthcare sector are far-reaching. Healthcare providers, institutions, and insurers can assist keep the healthcare system financially stable and ensure patients get the care they need by taking measures to reduce fraud and abuse.

Coverage for patient services and waivers

In order to give the highest standard of care to patients, healthcare professionals need an in-depth familiarity with the various insurance plans on the market. When delivering medical care, familiarity with each insurance company's policies and procedures is essential. To receive the best care possible, patients should familiarize themselves with their insurance plans and perks. Furthermore, due to their financial circumstances, certain patients may need financial assistance or waivers. In order to give the greatest treatment possible, it is crucial to be aware of these possibilities.

Patients and their families can rest easy knowing they are financially protected thanks to health insurance. Public health insurance, private health insurance, and insurance provided by one's work are just a few of the many options available to those in need of financial protection. Individuals or their employers may acquire private health insurance plans that provide financial protection against the costs associated with medical care. Medicare, Medicaid, and other similar programs are examples of government-sponsored insurance. Those who meet the program's age, income, or disability requirements are eligible for coverage. Insurance that is offered and paid for by an employer, either in whole or in part, is called employer-sponsored insurance.

Patients may benefit from having someone explain their insurance plan and its provisions to them. The patient is responsible for knowing the extent of their plan's coverage and any potential out-of-pocket expenses. Healthcare providers have a responsibility to their patients to check their insurance coverage and eligibility prior to offering any treatments.

Patients' financial situations may necessitate financial aid in specific scenarios. Patients who fulfill the program's income standards may be eligible for financial assistance from some healthcare providers. Low-income people and families may be eligible for healthcare coverage through government-sponsored programs like Medicaid.

Patients who lack health insurance or cannot pay for necessary medical care may be eligible for a waiver. Waivers for fees associated with specific medical procedures or treatments are sometimes made available by doctors and hospitals so that people can get the care they need without going into debt. In order to qualify for a waiver, patients often need to meet financial or residence requirements.

Healthcare practitioners cannot provide optimal treatment for their patients without a thorough understanding of insurance policies, patient financial assistance programs, and eligibility for waivers. Patients have a responsibility to learn about and comprehend all of their healthcare alternatives and costs. For patients to get the care they need without having to worry about how to pay for it, healthcare professionals must be well-versed on insurance plans and coverage.

Insurance types/third-party payers

Third-party payers and insurance policies play a crucial role in the healthcare financing system. Health insurance was created to shield individuals from the financial burden of paying for medical care out of pocket. Employers, the government, and private individuals can all offer health insurance to their employees.

HMOs, PPOs, EPOs, and POS plans are the most typical kinds of health insurance. HMOs, or health maintenance organizations, offer patients consistent costs for medical care. All healthcare needs must be coordinated through a patient's chosen primary care physician (PCP). In order to see a specialist, HMO members often need a recommendation from their primary care physician.

Healthcare services are also available at a flat charge through Preferred Provider Organizations (PPOs). Patients can see any specialist they want without a referral from their PCP, but they are not compelled to do so. PPOs give patients with access to a network of healthcare providers that charge reduced fees for their services. Patients have the option of seeing in-network or out-of-network providers, with the latter often incurring greater costs.

EPOs are similar to PPOs in that members are not obligated to choose a primary care physician (PCP). However, only healthcare providers in an EPO's network will be covered. Patients frequently bear the entire financial burden of treatment when seeking medical care from a healthcare professional who is not affiliated with their insurance provider's network.

POS plans are a hybrid between HMOs and PPOs. Patients must choose a primary care physician (PCP) and obtain referrals to specialists, but they have the option of paying more to access care from non-network providers.

Medicare and Medicaid are examples of government-funded insurance programs that act as third-party payers and cover qualified patients. Medicare is a government health insurance program for those 65 and up, or those with qualifying disabilities. Medicaid is a health insurance program for low-income individuals and families that is supported by the state.

Patients can also seek coverage from private insurance firms. These policies can be obtained alone or as part of an employer's benefits package. Individuals and families can find private insurance policies that match their specific needs in terms of coverage, price, and other factors.

Healthcare financing relies heavily on health insurance and other forms of third-party payment. In order to offer the best treatment possible for their patients and to ensure that they receive enough reimbursement for their services, healthcare practitioners must have a thorough understanding of the various insurance plans and third-party payers.

Financial terminology

The ability to effectively manage a healthcare organization's finances requires a solid grasp of financial terminology. In this chapter, we'll define a number of healthcare-specific financial concepts.

Revenue is one of the cornerstones of accounting, and it represents the money brought in by the healthcare business from services provided to patients, laboratory tests performed on those patients, and diagnostic imaging performed on those patients. The costs incurred by the organization in delivering healthcare services are referred to as expenses, another key financial word. All costs, both direct (employee pay and benefits) and indirect (rent, utilities, and supplies) are factored in.

Accounts receivable, which is money owed to the healthcare business by patients and insurance companies for services rendered, is another crucial financial term. In order to secure timely payment and minimize bad debt, healthcare organizations keep a tight eye on their accounts receivable.

Healthcare businesses employ financial ratios as another indicator of financial health alongside income, costs, and accounts receivable. The financial stability of a firm can be assessed using many metrics, such as the current ratio, which assesses the company's ability to fulfill its short-term financial obligations, and the debt-to-equity ratio, which quantifies the company's debt relative to its equity.

The term "budgeting" is also frequently heard in the context of healthcare finance. Budgeting is making predictions about income and expenditures and coming up with a strategy for allocating funds to meet desired outcomes. Creating a budget for each division of the healthcare company and changing it as necessary are both part of this process.

The financial performance of healthcare organizations is reported using a number of different financial statements in addition to the aforementioned words. The income statement details the company's earnings and expenditures during a given time frame, whereas the balance sheet depicts the company's financial status as of a given date. The cash flow statement details the cash received and spent by the business over a given time frame.

Healthcare personnel need a solid grasp of financial jargon in order to efficiently oversee the business side of things. This involves making sure money isn't wasted and that the business can keep running for the foreseeable future.

Understanding the monetary lingo used in healthcare administration is crucial. It helps healthcare companies manage their money better, get an accurate picture of their financial standing, and allocate resources wisely. All healthcare personnel, from receptionists to CEOs, need a firm grasp of the lingo used in finance to safeguard the long-term health of their respective institutions.

Patient account financial procedures

Financial procedures for patient accounts are the steps taken to manage the money side of patient care. Billing, collecting payments, handling insurance claims, and administering aid programs all fall under this category. In order to conduct financial transactions in a timely, accurate, and ethical manner, healthcare organizations need to have clear policies and processes in place. Various monetary processes associated with patient accounts will be covered here.

Billing

A patient's services are billed when an invoice or account statement is created for them. Prices for all healthcare-related services, including as consultations, exams, and procedures. Coding and charge capture, claim submission, and follow-up on unpaid claims are just a few of the many phases involved in the billing process. Health care providers and facilities rely heavily on billing as a revenue generator and a means of making consumers aware of their financial responsibilities.

Payment Collection

The term "payment collection" refers to the act of requesting and receiving payment from clients.

This entails getting money for things like co-pays, deductibles, and so on. You can pay in cash when you receive the service, send an invoice in the mail, or use an online payment gateway. In order to ensure that payments are collected on time and accurately, healthcare organizations need to have clear rules in place.

Insurance Claims Processing

Processing claims for payment from insurance providers is known as insurance claims processing. Insurance coverage verification, service pre-authorization, and claim submission are just a few of the processes in this procedure. In spite of the difficulties inherent in the process, medical facilities really must submit insurance claims in order to get paid for their services in a timely manner.

Financial Assistance Programs

Patients who are unable to pay for healthcare treatments out of pocket may qualify for one of the many financial assistance programs offered by healthcare providers. Sliding scales, charity care, and government-sponsored programs like Medicaid and Medicare are all examples of what can fall under this category. In order to ensure that financial aid programs are managed fairly and ethically, healthcare organizations need to have clear regulations in place.

It is imperative for healthcare companies to implement financial procedures for patient accounts to ensure that all monetary transactions are handled in a timely, accurate, and ethical manner. To make sure patients get the care they need and healthcare providers get the money they need to run, there must be well-defined policies and procedures in place for billing, payment collection, insurance claims processing, and financial assistance programs. Healthcare companies can deliver high-quality service while simultaneously retaining financial viability through the use of efficient patient account finance operations.

Billing/collections

Healthcare management includes billing and collections. The term "billing" is used to describe the process of creating bills for services provided and sending them to patients, insurance companies, or other third-party payers. The term "collections" refers to the practice of requesting and receiving payment for these services from patients or their insurers. For healthcare facilities to remain financially stable and provide the treatment their patients require, efficient billing and collections procedures are vital.

Scheduling Appointments and Health Information Management

Scheduling visits for patients and keeping track of their medical records are two of the most important but often overlooked aspects of working in healthcare. Appointment management and patient data storage are the primary topics of this section. Appointment scheduling is the process of planning appointments for patients in a timely and orderly manner, whereas health information management includes the storage and maintenance of patient records, such as EHRs, filing systems, and charting procedures. Here, we'll discuss some of the most useful methods for keeping track of patients' visits and medical records.

Scheduling appointments

Appointment scheduling is a crucial component of running a successful medical practice, clinic, or hospital. It requires the integration of patient requirements, healthcare provider availability, and resource optimization. Patient satisfaction, wait times, and healthcare personnel' productivity can all benefit from a well-organized appointment scheduling system. In this article, we'll go over the fundamentals of scheduling appointments, such as the various scheduling systems available, how to set up reminders for scheduled events, and general scheduling best practices.

Appropriate scheduling system selection is a crucial step in the appointment-setting process. Open-access scheduling, double-booking scheduling, cluster scheduling, and wave scheduling are just a few of the many scheduling methods out there. Appointments can be made for the same or following day under an open access scheduling system. Two patients are booked into the same appointment time slot, with the possibility that one of them will have to wait longer than the other. Appointments in a cluster scheduling system are planned at the same time, while patients in a wave scheduling system are scheduled in waves at the same time. A healthcare facility's needs, healthcare practitioners' availability, and patients' preferences will all factor into the decision of which scheduling system to use.

Using appointment reminders is also a crucial part of appointment scheduling. Improved patient outcomes and lower healthcare expenses are both possible with the use of appointment reminders. Appointment reminders can come in many forms, such as prerecorded phone calls, text messages, and emails. The healthcare center and its patients will jointly decide on the best appointment reminder system.

Appointment scheduling and appointment reminders are two examples of scheduling best practices that can increase both patient happiness and healthcare practitioners' productivity. Appointment length, healthcare provider, and follow-up visits are just a few of the factors that should be taken into account while scheduling patients. Appointments should be scheduled with the proper urgency, and patients should be prioritized based on the severity of their disease.

Appointment scheduling is a crucial component of running a successful medical practice, clinic, or hospital. Better patient outcomes, lower healthcare costs, and more efficient healthcare delivery are all possible when healthcare practitioners use the right scheduling system, remind patients of their appointments, and follow other best scheduling practices.

Electronic health records (EHRs)

Information like as a patient's medical history, diagnosis, prescriptions, treatment plan, immunization dates, laboratory test results, and more can be found in an EHR. Electronic health records (EHRs) are intended to make patient information easily accessible to authorized healthcare practitioners in order to improve the quality and safety of patient care. The guidelines for EHR deployment, as well as the pros and cons of EHRs, their impact on healthcare organizations, and more will be covered here.

Benefits of EHRs

The increased focus on patient safety is a major advantage of EHRs. Medical mistakes like prescribing the wrong drug or delivering an anti-allergy treatment can be avoided with the help of electronic health records (EHRs). Medical professionals can use EHRs to track their patients' impending appointments for preventative screenings and diagnostics.

By lowering the amount of time spent on administrative duties like filling out paperwork and searching for patient records, EHRs can also improve the quality and efficiency of healthcare. As an added bonus, electronic health records can make it easier for doctors and nurses to talk to one another, leading to better care coordination.

Challenges of EHRs

The use of electronic health records (EHRs) has many advantages, but it also has its drawbacks. The high price tag of putting this plan into action is a major obstacle. The acquisition, installation, and training of an electronic health record system can be financially burdensome for healthcare providers. When it comes to federal and state laws like HIPAA, healthcare providers have an additional responsibility to ensure that their EHR system is in full compliance.

One more thing that could go wrong with EHRs is a security compromise. Electronic health records (EHRs) include private patient information, thus healthcare providers must take precautions to safeguard it. Firewalls, encryption, and other forms of access restriction are all part of this strategy.

Impact on Healthcare Organizations

Electronic health records have had a major effect on the healthcare industry. They have increased the effectiveness of healthcare delivery while also enhancing its quality and patient safety. Better health outcomes for patients may result from the increased communication and collaboration made possible by EHRs.

However, EHR implementation can be a massive task for hospitals and other healthcare facilities. Healthcare firms must invest heavily in EHRs and make sure their personnel is trained to use the system effectively. In addition, electronic health records (EHRs) need regular upkeep and updates to function properly.

Standards for EHR Implementation

To guarantee the efficiency and safety of EHRs, the federal government has set requirements for their deployment. Included in these guidelines is the Meaningful Use program, which offers financial incentives to healthcare providers who can prove they are making good use of their electronic health record system to advance the quality of patient care.

In addition, the EHR standards for data interchange and interoperability have been established by the Office of the National Coordinator for Health Information Technology (ONC). It is crucial that healthcare practitioners and organizations be able to exchange patient information, and these standards guarantee that electronic health record systems can connect with one another.

Electronic health records, or EHRs, have several advantages for both healthcare providers and their patients. However, healthcare organizations must ensure they are in accordance with state and federal legislation and standards for EHR adoption, which may be a substantial endeavor in and of itself. The quality of care provided to patients can be enhanced by healthcare organizations if they give due consideration to the advantages and disadvantages of EHRs and adopt them with forethought and strategy.

Types of filing systems

There are a number of different file systems used to organize patient records and other paperwork in the field of health information management. A company's filing system should be tailored to its specific requirements, the data it stores, and the resources it has at its disposal. Here we'll look at some of the most popular healthcare recordkeeping methods.

Alphabetical filing system

This style of medical record keeping is by far the most popular. Files are organized in alphabetical order by the patient's last name in an alphabetical filing system. This approach is straightforward and well-suited to clinics with a modest patient load. However, larger businesses with a greater number of patient records may find it challenging to handle.

Numeric filing system

Patient files in a numeric filing system each have their own numerical identifier. The records are sorted numerically based on this code. For healthcare facilities with a lot of paperwork, numerical filing systems are a good option. However, it might be challenging to manage if the company experiences a high rate of employee turnover.

Subjective filing system

A subjective filing system classifies documents according to their perceived relevance rather than any objective criteria. Organizations in the healthcare industry that deal with multiple medical subspecialties would benefit greatly from this method. However, it can be difficult to administer because it necessitates meticulous record-keeping to prevent redundant entries.

The terminal digit filing system is analogous to the numerical filing system, but with a few key differences. The last two digits of a given number are used to categorize data in this system. A document with the identifier 12345 would, for instance, be put under the 45 heading. Large healthcare providers with a lot of paperwork would benefit greatly from this solution. It lessens the possibility of misfiled documents and speeds up the time it takes to retrieve them.

Geographic filing system

Geographic filing organizes patient files according to where they were created. Multiple-location healthcare providers can benefit greatly from this method. However, it can be challenging to manage if there are many mobile patients in the business.

There are good and bad aspects to every type of filing system. A company's filing system should be tailored to its specific requirements, the data it stores, and the resources it has at its disposal. Regardless of the method selected, meticulous labeling and filing of information is essential for speedy access in an emergency.

It is essential to think about the type of charting approach utilized to document patient information in addition to selecting the proper file system. In the following part, we'll talk about the many healthcare charting options now in use.

Types of charting methods

Different healthcare facilities use a variety of charting systems to collect and organize patient data. Information on patients can be recorded in a variety of formats, including paper and digital ones. Accurately recording and organizing vital patient data in a way that facilitates quick retrieval and sharing among healthcare personnel is a hallmark of efficient charting practices.

Some of the most widespread healthcare charting approaches include the following:

Narrative Charting

Free-form narrative writing is used to document a patient's history. Notes are broken down into the four categories of SOAP format: subjective, objective, assessment, and plan. This strategy is helpful for patients with complex medical histories or who will be staying in a long-term care facility, as it gives a complete record of the care they have received.

Problem-Oriented Medical Record (POMR)

The Problem-Oriented Medical Record (POMR) system is a way of keeping track of patient data based on the presenting medical issue. There are four parts to this approach: a database, a list of issues, a treatment plan, and a log of results. Providers may gain a deeper comprehension of the patient's medical issues and treatment outcomes with the aid of the POMR method, which takes a more targeted approach to charting.

Source-Oriented Medical Record (SOMR)

The SOMR is a conventional approach to diagramming that divides data into pieces according to its origin. When compared to other approaches, this one is less organized and could make it harder to retrieve the data at a later date.

Electronic Health Record (EHR)

Electronic health records (EHRs) are digital copies of patient records that include information such as a patient's medical history, diagnostic test results, medications, allergies, and more. Electronic health records (EHRs) facilitate better communication and collaboration between medical professionals, lessen the likelihood of medical mistakes, and give consumers more control over their own health data.

Problem List Charting

The patient's list of symptoms serves as the focal point of the charting in this approach. Keeping track of individual issues, evaluations, and fixes is essential. The patient's medical history can be summarized quickly and easily using this method.

Instead of recording even the smallest changes in a patient's state, "charting by exception" (CBE) only records those that are clinically important. Time is conserved, duplication is reduced, and it may be simpler to spot shifts in a patient's health when using this approach.

Flow Sheet Charting

Documenting particular patient data such as vital signs, laboratory results, and other information on a standard sheet is called flow sheet charting. When new information is available, it is added to the flowchart. This strategy is helpful for monitoring a patient's development over time and spotting unusual fluctuations promptly.

The care context, the patient's condition, and the provider's preferences all play a role in deciding which charting style is best. Electronic health records (EHRs) have completely changed the way medical charts are kept because of technological advancements. No matter what system is chosen, the most important thing is that patient records are accurate and comprehensive.

Secret Keys

It's not easy to get yourself ready to take the Certified Medical Assistant (CMA) exam. However, if you go into it with the appropriate frame of mind, you may find it to be rather gratifying. In this supplementary chapter, we'll reveal three strategies for passing the CMA exam with flying colors. This is the key:

Plan Big, Study Small And Smart

One of the most important keys to success in any endeavor, including passing the CMA (Certified Medical Assistant) exam, is to plan big, study small, and study smart. In other words, set ambitious goals for yourself, break them down into smaller, manageable steps, and use effective study strategies to maximize your learning and retention.

Plan Big: Set Ambitious Goals

The first step to achieving any goal is to set a clear and specific objective. For the CMA exam, this means identifying your target score and the date by which you want to achieve it. You should also break down the exam into its various sections (clinical, administrative, and general), and set specific targets for each section. Finally, create a study schedule that allocates sufficient time for each section, and factor in some extra time for review and practice exams.

Study Small

Once you have set your goals, it is time to break them down into smaller, more manageable steps. This can involve creating a study plan that focuses on one section at a time, or breaking each section down into smaller topics or themes. For example, in the clinical section, you may want to focus on one body system at a time (such as the cardiovascular system, respiratory system, or musculoskeletal system), or one type of procedure (such as venipuncture, electrocardiography, or wound care). Breaking the material down in this way can make it easier to focus on and absorb.

Study Smart

Use Effective Learning Strategies

Finally, to make the most of your study time and maximize your retention of the material, it is important to use effective learning strategies. Some key strategies for CMA exam prep include:

Active learning

Rather than simply reading and re-reading the material, actively engage with it by taking notes, asking questions, and applying it to real-world scenarios.

Practice exams: Take advantage of practice exams (available through various online resources and study materials) to familiarize yourself with the format of the exam, assess your strengths and weaknesses, and identify areas in need of further review.

Mnemonic devices

Use mnemonic devices (such as acronyms, rhymes, or visual associations) to help you remember key concepts or information.

Group study

Consider studying with a group of fellow CMA exam candidates, as this can provide additional support, motivation, and opportunities for discussion and practice.

Personalized study: Tailor your study approach to your individual learning style and preferences. For example, if you are a visual learner, consider using diagrams, charts, and videos to help you understand the material.

How To Make Studying Productive

Studying is an essential part of learning, and it can often be a challenging and overwhelming task. With so much information to absorb and retain, it can be easy to get distracted, lose focus, and end up feeling frustrated and unproductive. However, by implementing some effective study techniques, you can maximize your study time, increase your productivity, and achieve better results. In this section we will explore some strategies for making your studying more productive and efficient.

Create a study schedule

The first step to making your studying more productive is to create a study schedule. This involves setting aside dedicated time for studying and breaking it down into smaller, manageable sessions. By doing this, you can ensure that you are covering all the necessary material, avoid cramming sessions, and reduce stress and overwhelm.

When creating a study schedule, it is essential to take into account your individual learning style, work schedule, and other commitments. For instance, if you work during the day, you may need to schedule your study sessions in the evenings or on weekends. You may also need to consider your attention span and break up your study time into smaller, focused sessions, rather than long, continuous ones.

Eliminate distractions

One of the biggest challenges to productive studying is distractions. Whether it's social media, emails, or other notifications, distractions can quickly derail your focus and reduce your productivity. To avoid distractions, you may need to disconnect from the internet or use apps that block social media and other non-study related websites. You can also set aside a specific time for checking emails and messages, and avoid multitasking during your study sessions.

Use active learning strategies

Active learning is an effective way of retaining information and making your studying more productive. Active learning entails actively engaging with the subject matter, as opposed to adopting a passive approach of merely reading or listening. Some active learning strategies include:

Writing notes

Writing notes can help you remember information, organize your thoughts, and identify key points. You can also use different colors, highlighters, and symbols to make your notes more visually appealing and memorable.

Summarizing

Summarizing involves condensing the information into a few sentences or bullet points. This can help you identify the main ideas and reinforce your understanding of the material.

Practice questions

Practicing questions can help you apply your knowledge and identify any gaps in your understanding. You can also use practice questions to simulate exam conditions and improve your test-taking skills.

Mind mapping

Mind mapping involves creating a visual representation of the material, using diagrams, images, and keywords. This can help you see the connections between different concepts and reinforce your understanding.

Take breaks

Taking breaks is an essential part of making your studying more productive. When you take breaks, you give your brain time to rest and recharge, which can improve your concentration and retention. However, it is essential to take effective breaks, which means stepping away from your study material and engaging in a different activity. You can take a walk, listen to music, meditate, or do some light exercise.

Stay organized

Staying organized can help you make the most of your study time and reduce stress. This involves keeping your study materials in order, prioritizing your tasks, and breaking down your goals into manageable steps. You can use apps, calendars, and to-do lists to help you stay organized and on track.

Practice The Right Way

Practice is a crucial part of preparing for the CMA exam. However, it's not just about practicing as much as possible but also practicing the right way. In this bonus chapter, we will discuss the key strategies for practicing the right way to maximize your chances of success on the CMA exam.

Focus on Weak Areas

One of the most important things to keep in mind while practicing is to focus on your weak areas. It's easy to get comfortable with the topics you already know, but it's important to identify and work on the areas where you need more practice. This can be done by taking mock exams, quizzes, and reviewing past exam results. Once you know your weak areas, you can create a study plan that prioritizes those topics.

Mimic Real Exam Conditions

To prepare yourself for the real CMA exam, it's important to practice under similar conditions. Set aside a specific time and space for your practice sessions, and make sure you're taking them seriously. Eliminate all distractions, including your phone and social media, and try to create an environment that mimics the real exam setting.

Use Practice Questions and Mock Exams

Practice questions and mock exams are essential tools for preparing for the CMA exam. They give you a chance to test your knowledge, identify weak areas, and become familiar with the format of the exam. Make sure to use a variety of sources for practice questions and mock exams to get a well-rounded view of the exam. You can find practice questions and mock exams in textbooks, review courses, and online resources.

Review and Analyze Results

After completing practice questions and mock exams, it's important to review and analyze your results. This will help you identify your weak areas and give you an idea of where to focus your study efforts. Make sure to read the explanations for incorrect answers and use them to guide your future study sessions.

Don't Just Memorize

While memorization is an important part of studying, it's not enough to just memorize facts and formulas. You need to understand the concepts behind them to truly succeed on the CMA exam. Take the time to read and understand the material, and practice applying it to real-world scenarios.

Time Yourself

Time management is a key factor in success on the CMA exam. It's important to practice answering questions under time pressure to simulate the real exam. Set a timer for each practice session and try to answer questions within the allotted time frame. This will help you get comfortable with the pace of the exam and ensure that you can complete it within the given time.

Take Breaks

While practicing is important, it's also important to take breaks. Studying for extended periods of time without a break can lead to burnout and decreased productivity. Take short breaks every hour or so to give your brain a chance to rest and recharge. This will help you stay focused and engaged during your practice sessions.

Multiple Choice Questions

Chapter 1

1. **What is the term for a condition in which there is an insufficient amount of red blood cells or hemoglobin in the blood?**

    A) Anemia

    B) Arthritis

    C) Asthma

    D) Appendicitis

2. **Which of the following is a non-communicable disease?**

    A) Tuberculosis

    B) Influenza

    C) Cancer

    D) Malaria

3. **Which of the following is not considered one of the vital signs?**

    A) Blood pressure

    B) Temperature

    C) Respiration rate

    D) Body mass index

4. **Which of the following is the correct order of the phases of the nursing process?**

    A) Assessment, planning, implementation, evaluation

    B) Planning, assessment, implementation, evaluation

    C) Evaluation, assessment, planning, implementation

D) Assessment, implementation, planning, evaluation

5. **Which of the following is not a type of nursing intervention?**

   A) Administering medication

   B) Educating the patient

   C) Ordering diagnostic tests

   D) Providing emotional support

6. **Which of the following is not a characteristic of evidence-based practice?**

   A) Use of the best available evidence

   B) Incorporation of patient preferences

   C) Use of intuition and personal experience

   D) Consideration of clinical expertise

7. **What is the term for the process of communicating information about a patient's care to another healthcare provider?**

   A) Consultation

   B) Referral

   C) Transfer of care

   D) Handoff

8. **Which of the following is not a type of healthcare setting?**

   A) Acute care hospital

   B) Long-term care facility

   C) Private physician's office

   D) Retail pharmacy

9. **Which of the following is not a component of cultural competence?**

   A) Awareness of one's own cultural beliefs and biases

   B) Knowledge of the patient's culture

   C) Ability to speak the patient's language

   D) Respect for the patient's beliefs and values

10. **Which of the following is not a type of patient assessment?**

   A) Comprehensive assessment

   B) Focused assessment

   C) Functional assessment

   D) Diagnostic assessment

11. **What is the term for a set of rules or principles that govern conduct?**

   A) Ethics

   B) Morals

   C) Values

   D) Beliefs

12. **Which of the following is not a type of healthcare law?**

   A) Criminal law

   B) Civil law

   C) Administrative law

   D) Medical law

13. **Which of the following is not a type of healthcare professional?**

   A) Physician

   B) Nurse

   C) Dentist

   D) Pharmacist

14. **Which of the following is not a type of healthcare insurance?**

   A) Medicare

   B) Medicaid

   C) Social Security

   D) Private insurance

15. **What is the term for the process of examining healthcare data to improve quality of care and reduce costs?**

   A) Utilization review

B) Quality improvement

C) Risk management

D) Peer review

Chapter 2

1. **What is the purpose of an electronic health record (EHR)?**

    A) To store paper-based medical records.

    B) To improve the quality and safety of patient care.

    C) To reduce the need for healthcare providers.

    D) To eliminate the need for medical coding.

2. **What is the difference between a subjective and objective assessment in patient charting?**

    A) Subjective assessment is based on facts while objective assessment is based on feelings.

    B) Subjective assessment is based on symptoms reported by the patient while objective assessment is based on physical examination.

    C) Subjective assessment is based on the healthcare provider's opinion while objective assessment is based on the patient's opinion.

    D) Subjective assessment is based on laboratory results while objective assessment is based on vital signs.

3. **Which of the following is a disadvantage of a paper-based medical record system?**

    A) It is less expensive than an electronic health record system.

    B) It is easier to share records with other healthcare providers.

    C) It can be difficult to read and interpret handwritten notes.

    D) It allows for easier tracking of patient data over time.

4. **Which filing system organizes medical records according to the patient's condition or disease?**

    A) Alphabetical

    B) Numeric

    C) Subject

    D) Chronological

5. **Which charting method uses problem lists, care plans, and progress notes to track a patient's care?**

   A) SOAP notes

   B) Focus charting

   C) Charting by exception

   D) Case management

6. **Which of the following is a benefit of an electronic health record system?**

   A) It reduces the risk of errors due to illegible handwriting.

   B) It eliminates the need for healthcare providers.

   C) It is less expensive than a paper-based medical record system.

   D) It does not require training for healthcare providers.

7. **Which type of scheduling system assigns each patient a specific appointment time?**

   A) Open access

   B) Wave scheduling

   C) Double booking

   D) Time-specific scheduling

8. **Which of the following is a disadvantage of double booking?**

   A) It allows for more efficient use of healthcare provider's time.

   B) It can result in long wait times for patients.

   C) It does not allow for same-day appointments.

   D) It eliminates the need for appointment reminders.

9. **Which type of scheduling system allows patients to be seen on a first-come, first-served basis?**

   A) Open access

   B) Wave scheduling

   C) Double booking

   D) Cluster scheduling

10. **Which of the following is a disadvantage of open access scheduling?**

    A) It can result in long wait times for patients.

    B) It does not allow for same-day appointments.

    C) It requires patients to schedule appointments far in advance.

    D) It eliminates the need for appointment reminders.

11. **Which of the following is an advantage of a computerized appointment scheduling system?**

    A) It is less expensive than a paper-based system.

    B) It allows for easier scheduling of follow-up appointments.

    C) It eliminates the need for appointment reminders.

    D) It is not affected by power outages.

12. **Which of the following is an example of an electronic communication tool used in healthcare?**

    A) Fax machine

    B) Phone

    C) Email

    D) None of the above

13. **Which of the following is a disadvantage of telemedicine?**

    A) It is less convenient for patients than traditional office visits

    B) It can be more expensive than traditional office visits

    C) It is not as effective for remote patient monitoring as other methods

    D) It requires specialized equipment and technical expertise

14. **Which of the following is a type of electronic health record (EHR)?**

    A) Fax machine

    B) Paper chart

    C) Spreadsheet

    D) Patient portal

15. **Which of the following is a benefit of using electronic health records (EHRs)?**

    A) They are less secure than paper records

B) They are more time-consuming to use than paper records

C) They improve communication and coordination between healthcare providers

D) They are more prone to errors than paper records

Chapter 3

1. **What is the process of recording a patient's medical history?**

    A) Physical exam

    B) Diagnosis

    C) Assessment

    D) Medical interview

2. **Which of the following is NOT a component of the SOAP note?**

    A) Subjective

    B) Objective

    C) Assessment

    D) Plan

3. **Which of the following is a tool used to assess a patient's pain level?**

    A) Blood pressure monitor

    B) Pulse oximeter

    C) Pain scale

    D) Thermometer

4. **Which of the following is NOT a vital sign?**

    A) Blood pressure

    B) Heart rate

    C) Respiratory rate

    D) Body temperature

5. **What is the purpose of auscultation in a physical exam?**

    A) To measure blood pressure

    B) To listen to the sounds of the body

C) To assess reflexes

D) To test vision

6. **Which of the following is an example of a non-invasive diagnostic test?**

    A) CT scan

    B) X-ray

    C) MRI

    D) Ultrasound

7. **What is the process of obtaining a tissue sample for testing called?**

    A) Biopsy

    B) Autopsy

    C) Echocardiogram

    D) Electroencephalogram

8. **Which of the following is a diagnostic test used to evaluate brain function?**

    A) EKG

    B) EEG

    C) CT scan

    D) MRI

9. **Which of the following is NOT a common type of medical imaging?**

    A) CT scan

    B) MRI

    C) PET scan

    D) Pap smear

10. **What is the purpose of a urinalysis?**

    A) To diagnose anemia

    B) To evaluate kidney function

    C) To assess lung function

    D) To diagnose a heart attack

11. What is the process of withdrawing blood for testing called?

    A) Biopsy

    B) Phlebotomy

    C) Electroencephalogram

    D) Endoscopy

12. Which of the following is NOT a type of medical specimen?

    A) Blood

    B) Urine

    C) Stool

    D) Hair

13. What is the purpose of a Pap smear?

    A) To evaluate kidney function

    B) To diagnose a heart attack

    C) To screen for cervical cancer

    D) To monitor blood glucose levels

14. Which of the following is a type of diagnostic test used to evaluate heart function?

    A) EEG

    B) EKG

    C) CT scan

    D) PET scan

15. What is the process of visualizing the inside of the body using an endoscope called?

    A) Biopsy

    B) Autopsy

    C) Endoscopy

    D) Echocardiogram

Chapter 4

1. **Which of the following is not a purpose of medical coding?**

   A) Facilitating communication between healthcare providers

   B) Ensuring compliance with legal and regulatory requirements

   C) Facilitating payment and reimbursement

   D) Diagnosing medical conditions

2. **What is the purpose of the ICD-10-CM coding system?**

   A) To classify diseases and injuries

   B) To report medical procedures and services

   C) To identify healthcare providers

   D) To manage patient appointments

3. **What is the purpose of the CPT coding system?**

   A) To classify diseases and injuries

   B) To report medical procedures and services

   C) To identify healthcare providers

   D) To manage patient appointments

4. **Which of the following is a type of coding used to report medical procedures and services?**

   A) ICD-10-CM

   B) HCPCS

   C) CDT

   D) DSM-5

5. **What is the purpose of modifier codes in medical coding?**

   A) To indicate the location of a medical service

   B) To indicate the severity of a medical condition

   C) To provide additional information about a medical service

   D) To indicate the duration of a medical treatment

6. **Which of the following is a type of modifier code?**

   A) HCPCS

   B) CPT

   C) ICD-10-CM

   D) HCPCS Level II

7. **What is the purpose of the National Correct Coding Initiative (NCCI)?**

   A) To ensure consistency in medical coding

   B) To provide training for medical coders

   C) To certify medical coders

   D) To regulate medical coding fees

8. **What is the purpose of the Healthcare Common Procedure Coding System (HCPCS)?**

   A) To classify diseases and injuries

   B) To report medical procedures and services

   C) To identify healthcare providers

   D) To manage patient appointments

9. **Which of the following is a type of HCPCS code?**

   A) Level I

   B) Level II

   C) ICD-10-CM

   D) CPT

10. **What is the purpose of the Centers for Medicare and Medicaid Services (CMS)?**

    A) To provide healthcare services

    B) To regulate healthcare providers

    C) To administer government healthcare programs

    D) To accredit healthcare facilities

11. **What is the purpose of the Resource-Based Relative Value Scale (RBRVS)?**

    A) To determine medical necessity for procedures and services

B) To set reimbursement rates for procedures and services

C) To regulate healthcare providers

D) To classify diseases and injuries

12. What is the purpose of a medical claim form?

A) To report medical procedures and services to insurance companies

B) To classify diseases and injuries for research purposes

C) To identify healthcare providers for government programs

D) To manage patient appointments

13. Which of the following is a type of medical claim form?

A) UB-04

B) CMS-1500

C) ICD-10-CM

D) CPT

14. What is the purpose of a remittance advice?

A) To report medical procedures and services to insurance companies

B) To classify diseases and injuries for research purposes

C) To provide payment information to healthcare providers

D) To manage patient appointments

15. Which of the following is a type of remittance advice?

A) EOB

B) EOC

C) EOP

D) EON

Chapter 5

1. What is the purpose of medical coding?

A) To ensure patient privacy

B) To track patient demographics

C) To facilitate insurance billing and reimbursement

D) To provide patient care instructions

2. **Which organization is responsible for maintaining and updating the ICD-10-CM code set?**

   A) American Medical Association (AMA)

   B) Centers for Medicare and Medicaid Services (CMS)

   C) World Health Organization (WHO)

   D) National Center for Health Statistics (NCHS)

3. **What is the difference between ICD and CPT coding?**

   A) ICD codes are used for procedures, while CPT codes are used for diagnoses.

   B) ICD codes are used for diagnoses, while CPT codes are used for procedures.

   C) ICD codes are used for outpatient services, while CPT codes are used for inpatient services.

   D) ICD codes are used for mental health services, while CPT codes are used for physical health services.

4. **What is the purpose of modifier codes in medical coding?**

   A) To indicate a change in the patient's condition

   B) To indicate a change in the provider's specialty

   C) To indicate a change in the procedure performed

   D) To indicate a change in the patient's insurance coverage

5. **Which of the following code sets is used to report medical services and procedures in outpatient settings?**

   A) ICD-10-PCS

   B) CPT

   C) HCPCS Level II

   D) NDC

6. **What is the purpose of the National Correct Coding Initiative (NCCI)?**

   A) To prevent fraudulent billing practices

   B) To promote consistent coding practices

C) To establish payment rates for medical services

D) To determine medical necessity for services

7. **Which of the following is a type of HCPCS Level II code?**

   A) E/M codes

   B) J codes

   C) V codes

   D) G codes

8. **Which of the following is a type of CPT code?**

   A) Category II codes

   B) Category III codes

   C) Category IV codes

   D) Category V codes

9. **What is the purpose of an ABN (Advance Beneficiary Notice) in medical coding?**

   A) To inform the patient of their diagnosis

   B) To inform the patient of the cost of their care

   C) To inform the patient of their treatment options

   D) To inform the patient of their insurance coverage

10. **Which of the following is an example of a Category I CPT code?**

    A) 99201

    B) 99281

    C) 96372

    D) G0101

11. **Which of the following is a type of ICD-10-CM code?**

    A) E/M codes

    B) HCPCS Level II codes

    C) V codes

    D) Z codes

12. **Which of the following is a type of modifier code?**

    A) Global Surgical Package modifier

    B) Evaluation and Management (E/M) modifier

    C) Diagnosis Pointer modifier

    D) Payment Adjustment modifier

13. **What is the purpose of a fee schedule in medical coding?**

    A) To determine the amount charged for a specific service

    B) To determine the amount reimbursed for a specific service

    C) To determine the patient's out-of-pocket expenses

    D) To determine the provider's overhead costs

14. **Which of the following is a type of NDC code?**

    A) J codes

    B) V codes

    C) Q codes

    D) 11-digit NDC codes

15. **Which of the following is a type of ICD-10-PCS code?**

    A) Category I codes

    B) Category II codes

    C) Category III codes

    D) Category IV codes

Answers

Chapter 1

1. A) Anemia
2. C) Cancer
3. D) Body mass index
4. A) Assessment, planning, implementation, evaluation
5. C) Ordering diagnostic tests
6. C) Use of intuition and personal experience
7. D) Handoff
8. D) Retail pharmacy
9. C) Ability to speak the patient's language
10. D) Diagnostic assessment
11. A) Ethics
12. D) Medical law
13. C) Dentist
14. C) Social Security
15. B) Quality improvement

Chapter 2

1. B) To improve the quality and safety of patient care.
2. B) Subjective assessment is based on symptoms reported by the patient while objective assessment is based on physical examination.
3. C) It can be difficult to read and interpret handwritten notes.

4. C) Subject.

5. B) Focus charting.

6. A) It reduces the risk of errors due to illegible handwriting.

7. D) Time-specific scheduling.

8. B) It can result in long wait times for patients.

9. A) Open access.

10. A) It can result in long wait times for patients.

11. B) It allows for easier scheduling of follow-up appointments.

12. C) Email.

13. D) It requires specialized equipment and technical expertise.

14. D) Patient portal.

15. C) They improve communication and coordination between healthcare providers.

Chapter 3

1. D) Medical interview

2. C) Assessment

3. C) Pain scale

4. D) Body temperature

5. B) To listen to the sounds of the body

6. D) Ultrasound

7. A) Biopsy

8. B) EEG

9. D) Pap smear

10. B) To evaluate kidney function

11. B) Phlebotomy

12. D) Hair

13. C) To screen for cervical cancer

14. B) EKG

15. C) Endoscopy

Chapter 4

1. D) Diagnosing medical conditions

2. A) To classify diseases and injuries

3. B) To report medical procedures and services

4. B) HCPCS

5. C) To provide additional information about a medical service

6. D) HCPCS Level II

7. A) To ensure consistency in medical coding

8. B) To report medical procedures and services

9. B) Level II

10. C) To administer government healthcare programs

11. B) To set reimbursement rates for procedures and services

12. A) To report medical procedures and services to insurance companies

13. B) CMS-1500

14. C) To provide payment information to healthcare providers

15. A) EOB

Chapter 5

1. C) To facilitate insurance billing and reimbursement

2. D) National Center for Health Statistics (NCHS)

3. B) ICD codes are used for diagnoses, while CPT codes are used for procedures.

4. C) To indicate a change in the procedure performed

5. B) CPT

6. B) To promote consistent coding practices

7. B) J codes

8. A) Category II codes

9. B) To inform the patient of the cost of their care

10. A) 99201

11. D) Z codes

12. B) Evaluation and Management (E/M) modifier

13. B) To determine the amount reimbursed for a specific service

14. D) 11-digit NDC codes

15. A) Category I codes

Made in United States
Troutdale, OR
12/07/2023

15475607R00091